Your No Guilt Pregnancy Plan

Your No Guilt Pregnancy Plan

REBECCA SCHILLER

PENGUIN LIFE

AN IMPRINT OF

PENGUIN BOOKS

PENGUIN LIFE

UK | USA | Canada | Ireland | Australia
India | New Zealand | South Africa

Penguin Life is part of the Penguin Random House group of companies
whose addresses can be found at global.penguinrandomhouse.com.

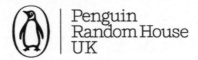

First published 2018
001

The information in this book has been compiled by way of general guidance in relation to the specific
subjects addressed. It is not a substitute and not to be relied on for medical, healthcare, pharmaceutical or
other professional advice on specific circumstances and in specific locations. Please consult your GP
before changing, stopping or starting any medical treatment. So far as the author is aware the
information given is correct and up to date as at January 2018. Practice, laws and regulations all change, and the
reader should obtain up-to-date professional advice on any such issues. The author and publishers disclaim,
as far as the law allows, any liability arising directly or indirectly from the use, or misuse, of the
information contained in this book.

Set in 13.5/16 pt Garamond MT Std
Typeset by Jouve (UK), Milton Keynes
Printed in Great Britain by Clays Ltd, St Ives plc

A CIP catalogue record for this book is available from the British Library

ISBN: 978–0–241–31580–4

www.greenpenguin.co.uk

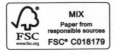

For Sofya and Arthur and the wonderful
world I want for you.

Contents

Introduction

I have been a mother for 8 wonderful and terrifying years. Motherhood has changed, exposed and expanded me. It has taken from me and offered back so much more – things I'm still scrabbling around in the dust for, trying to fit them into my understanding of who the hell I am and what I want to be. Pregnancy, birth and parenting have given me opportunities beyond the profound and simple wonder of making and getting to know my children. I've learned more about myself than at any other time in my life – things I am brilliant at, the many, many things I need to work on and what I need to just let go of and watch float away.

I've made the kind of friends who would walk over Lego pieces in bare feet for me – smiling encouragingly and carrying a gin and tonic. I've created 2 unique humans whom I can claim at least 50 per cent of the credit for, and discovered a flesh-eating virus of love for them that somehow leaves me both emptier and so much fuller than before. I've grown into my body and, thanks to a new kind of respect for it, I feel more comfortable in it. It has been a joy-filled, horizon-expanding, riot of a ride in so many ways, for me and for the people who will tell their stories in the pages that follow.

But for each of us, the journey to today hasn't always been a simple one. There have been contradictions, doubt, difficult decisions and plenty of conflicting and oh-so-strongly opinionated advice. The presence of a bump seems to give the rest of the world permission to poke about in our personal decisions, comment on our bodies and tell us that we aren't allowed to do as we want. How we feel about our births can have a long-lasting positive or negative impact on how we feel about ourselves. The staggering changes to our minds, bodies, lives and relationships aren't properly acknowledged and we're encouraged to scoop ourselves up, back into our jeans and former lives as if nothing had altered.

In a world that puts a lot of pressure on mothers, but doesn't do a good job of trusting, valuing, supporting and nurturing us, it's time to start a revolution and insist on a better, deeper, more realistic and less guilt-filled way to prepare for pregnancy, birth and parenting.

Why do you need this book?

You need this book because becoming a parent is about so much more than heartburn, crowning and breast pumps (though I'll cover that stuff too). It's about huge leaps, amazing opportunities, difficult circumstances, adventures, laughs, tears and the unexpected in bucket-loads. It's about your whole life.

I think we've been preparing for motherhood in some strange and unhelpful ways. It is often reduced to a one-dimensional, goal-orientated exercise, complete with a contradictory barrage of opinions, too many 'must haves' and 'must dos' and the promise of a perfect birth, baby and parenting experience at the end. This can cause problems in 3 significant ways.

Planning for perfection is unrealistic and will almost always lead to crashing disappointment and guilt. The narrow goals we are told to aim for exclude many people, and can make a wonderful but normal, bumpy journey feel like a failure.

Becoming a parent means changes to our work, sex lives, relationships, body image, mental health and bank balance that can have huge implications for the way we live and how we feel. Yet most pregnancy books spend more time comparing our babies to the size of various fruits than teaching us how to cope with the things that really matter. Having the best possible experience of birth on your own terms is really important and achievable (more on that later), but it isn't everything. If you only make a birth plan and don't think about a bigger plan, then you've missed out on the chance to set yourself up as well as possible for the new world that awaits you on the other side.

Relying on the opinions of others can leave you feeling conflicted and unsure of who to trust. It can stop you listening to what you already know about your body, your life and your needs, and can plunge you into an overwhelming sea of information and arguments about what's best.

You need this book because perfection isn't real. You won't have a 'perfect' pregnancy, a 'perfect' birth or a 'perfect' baby and you won't be a 'perfect' mother, **and that's OK**. In these pages I'll make sure you stop trying for the impossible and learn how to find a better, more realistic set of goals that fit with who you are.

I'll help you prepare for your fabulously good-enough reality with unbiased information and an honest conversation about how to make this new life fit with your existing one. We're planning for much more than birth in these pages, and I'll talk you through creating your bespoke, guilt-free plan for pregnancy, birth and motherhood itself.

And while you'll be exploring the evidence, your options and rights, I'll also be supporting you to make decisions yourself and encouraging you to draw on your own expertise and life experience as well as that of your caregivers. I'll help you cut through all the contradictory crap that's out there and focus on what really matters – but I won't tell you what to do or second-guess how you might think or feel.

I hope it will help make these 9 months (and more) feel right for you – no matter what happens. It's the book I would like to have had on my bedside table 8 years ago. Here's to a book, a birth and a future with no guilt, no judgement and absolutely no bullshit.

Who is this book for?

You may have stumbled on this book, positive pregnancy test in hand, along with a huge pile of magazines and DVDs, in an attempt to get your head round this 'argh, I'm having a baby' feeling. It may well have been foisted on you by a friend or random woman on the street.

You might be a planner-extraordinaire who arranged for the book to be delivered well before conception, or indeed the partner, mother, friend or even the teenage son or daughter (yes, this book is for the whole family) of a super-planner, who is reading this under strict instruction and supervision.

Perhaps these pages are already covered with cracker crumbs, yoghurt smears and the odd crayon scribble as you attempt to wrestle them off Child Number One and spend 2 minutes thinking about how this next one is going to make its appearance. Come on little Bert, PUT MUMMY'S BOOK DOWN.

Whoever you are and however it has ended up in your hands, rest assured that this book is for you. It doesn't matter whether you have very clear ideas about what's right for you when it comes to childbirth or parenting, or you don't know how to begin finding out about the decisions you might want to make; either way this book is designed to be your faithful companion over the coming months.

At no point in the next 21 chapters will I tell you what to do or what you aren't allowed to do. I don't know you, your body, your baby, your history, your set-up, your hopes or your fears. I am not an expert on you. I have a sneaking suspicion that nobody else is either. You don't need to feel guilty for having different priorities or realities to me or anyone else. I won't try to cunningly sway you in a certain direction using subliminal messages. I promise I won't tell you what I would do in your situation or the terrible thing that my imaginary sister did that you should avoid at all costs. You are the boss.

From the moment you read this, and forever more, know that you matter very much; that you are the expert on yourself and that you get to be in charge at all times – even when some things are beyond your control. You remain the same complicated human being with your own needs, wants and lovely imperfections as you were before you also became a mother. It might be hard to squeeze the old you and this new you together, but you can, and it is OK to wobble while you try. You matter and I won't let you forget it.

How to read this book

I've divided the book into three parts: pregnancy (page 9), birth (page 113) and afterwards (page 255), to allow you to read about what feels relevant and right to you at the right time. Each part will take you through the key milestones you will experience, the decisions you'll want to make and the information you'll need to help you make these. You'll find a range of different stories from women along the way and, because I know that all this can feel daunting, I'll take you through carefully chosen exercises, tools and tips to break it down and help you work out what's important to you. And at the end of each chapter you'll find a handy checklist reminding you where the most important tips and exercises can be found.

Your Body

The 'Your Body' chapters will encourage you to feel good in your skin and offer some help if you don't. We'll focus on how you prepare your body for what's to come and on understanding how it works in labour, but I won't add to the pressure, body-shaming and woman-policing attitude that is out there. This is not about making your body into the perfect baby-carrying device. You still get to own, experience, live in and be in touch with your body – for your own sake. You still get to enjoy sex, if you want to, eat crisps, if you like them, watch box sets or run up snowy mountains as you go into labour, whichever takes your fancy, even drink the odd beer – if it feels safe for you.

Your Mind

The 'Your Mind' chapters are even more important. With increasing awareness that new mothers can struggle emotionally, I think we need more exercises for our mind and less focus on physical perfection. Together we will look at how pregnancy, birth and beyond might impact on your mental health, as well as the important role your mind plays in childbirth. I will give you suggestions to help you identify issues and develop coping strategies before, during and after birth. If you have a partner I'll suggest ways to be open and upfront with each other about your different parenting styles and understand how the ways that you were each parented might influence your behaviour. I want to help you iron out major parenting kinks in your relationship before you have a 3-month-old baby and a backlog of sleep deprivation.

Your Life

I know that pregnancy is just one part of your life, albeit a big one. So in the 'Your Life' chapters I'll talk about work, money and maternity leave. We'll think about your relationships with your partner, your mother, your family and your friends. Can you still fly in an aeroplane? How much do you need to change your life or put it on hold? I want to encourage you not to do as you are told but instead help you to develop the skills to look at the evidence and work it out for yourself.

Alongside this I'll encourage you to prioritize setting yourself realistic expectations, not unachievable goals. The 'Your Decisions' chapters will help you explore the options for pregnancy, childbirth and feeding your baby. I'll give you lots of accurate information and practical tips for all kinds of births. I'll aim to be your perfect, non-judgemental, knowledgeable friend. In other words, I'll be your handbag-size doula (more on doulas in Chapter 13).

This book has been designed to be easy-to-read, honest but reassuring, and I don't want to add to your growing to-do list or feelings of pressure. You can read it from cover to cover, using the checklists at the end of each chapter to work out which exercises and tips are important for you. In the last chapter you'll use all you've discovered to make your own plan for pregnancy, birth and the first weeks with your new baby.

If you tend to feel overwhelmed by lots of new information and choices, you can also read the book in bite-size chunks. To use it this way you might like to start at the very end of the book – Chapter 21 – which will tell you which parts of the book to read in your particular situation and will point you to the various pieces of information, exercises and resources that you will find useful. Using this planning chapter as your guide, you can pick and choose what to read and do, while making your own, very concrete, reassuring and guilt-free plan for motherhood on your own terms.

Need more information?

Scientific research, pregnancy recommendations, support groups, books, blogs and equipment are continually updated. So if you want to read more about anything referenced in this book you'll find the latest links and much more at www.rebeccaschiller.co.uk/noguilt.

Part 1

Pregnancy

Chapter 1

Timeline of 40 weeks of pregnancy

0–2

Your pregnancy is dated from the first day of your last period. You actually conceive in week 2, so you aren't really pregnant in weeks 0 and 1.

2–4

Some pregnancy tests can detect the HCG hormone from as early as 6 days before your period. Tests are so reliable that your doctor or midwife will probably rely on your home test result. If the test says 'pregnant', you almost certainly are.

A week or two after conception you might notice some pink discharge or light spotting. For a third of women this bleeding is an outward sign of the embryo implanting in the uterine wall.

4–6

It's early days, but you might start to notice your breasts feeling sensitive, heavy or painful. They may start to grow, and can enlarge by a couple of cup sizes by the end of your pregnancy.

You can alert your GP to your pregnancy now, so that you get on to your local midwifery team's books. You can also self-refer to a particular team of midwives or hospital if you prefer.

6–8

Morning sickness can start now. 80 per cent of women will feel nauseous during the first trimester and half will actually be sick. Sorry!

8–10

Your first appointment with your midwife is likely to happen now. More information on page 81. Remember you are entitled to paid time off for antenatal appointments.

You may be feeling really exhausted, particularly towards the end of the day. You'll probably find your energy returns in the second trimester.

10–12

If you are having a 12-week scan it will happen around now. Ensuring that this scan happens between 11 and 13 weeks plus 6 days into your pregnancy is important if you want to have screening for congenital abnormalities.

Food cravings and aversions are really common in pregnancy, particularly in the first trimester. I couldn't get enough cold custard and had a much sweeter tooth than usual – but your cravings will be different. See page 26 for guidance on foods to try to limit or avoid in pregnancy.

13–15

Hurrah for the second trimester! The general feeling of bleurgh should start to lift now and certainly by 16 weeks. For many women the following weeks are all glowing skin, glossy hair and radiance. For the rest of us it's still a bit of a slog – especially if you are in the minority who still feel unwell (see page 105 for information on severe sickness). However you are feeling, see page 33 for some gentle exercise and calming tips to help you connect with your changing body.

Telling friends and family? Many people wait until the first scan is done, but if you want to tell people earlier, go ahead. You know what's right for you.

16–18

If this is your second pregnancy, you may have been feeling your baby move for a few weeks. First-timers may start to feel tiny, bubble-like movements around now. If you have an anterior placenta (one that has attached to the front of your uterus rather than the back), this acts as a cushion and you might not feel anything for a while.

You will be offered a midwife appointment at 16 weeks. They may suggest listening to the foetal heart rate at this point.

19–22

Have you researched your local antenatal classes yet? Some get booked up early, so it's worth getting ahead of the game. Your midwife should be able to book you in for free classes through your local hospital or midwife team. Loads of private options are available too.

At 20 weeks you will be offered an anomaly scan. See page 89 for more info.

Braxton Hicks contractions, or practice contractions, will have been happening since about 7 weeks, but you may start to feel them now. Staying hydrated, emptying your bladder and easing off exercising can help. If you are breastfeeding an older baby or toddler you may notice that this brings on Braxton Hicks.

Your midwife will be offering to measure the height of the top of your uterus (fundal height). By 20 weeks it is about level with your belly button.

23–25

As the third trimester approaches, lots of people start to prepare for their baby's arrival in earnest. Get on the list for NCT nearly-new sales, and talk to friends with older babies and children, as you may be able to borrow much of what you need.

If you haven't decided where you'd like to give birth, have a look at Chapter 11 and visit the Which? Birth Choices site to get the lowdown on the facilities in your area.

Week 25 is the last week in which you can tell your employer about your pregnancy. If this is your first pregnancy you'll also be offered an antenatal check-up around now.

26–28

Insomnia is really common, and deeply annoying, in the third trimester. Physical exercise and calming meditation can really help. Chamomile tea and essential oils help some. Alternatively, stock up on books, renew your Netflix subscription and consider it as conditioning you for a newborn.

You will be offered an antenatal check-up around 28 weeks.

Your breasts may have started producing colostrum (see page 300) as early as 14 weeks, but you may notice it leaking now. Some women are leakers, others aren't, so if you don't see any signs of colostrum that doesn't mean it isn't there.

Start sleeping on your left side around now, as this can reduce the chance of having a stillbirth. Try to start the night off on your left and don't worry if you wake up in a different position.

29–32 Your uterus has grown and you'll feel the top of it about 10cm above your belly button. Braxton Hicks contractions may feel stronger, and if it's your second or third baby these can be really frequent. Women who have been through labour before often have lots of 'false alarms' (or practice runs) before the real thing.

29 weeks is the earliest you can start your 'ordinary maternity leave' (see page 55).

At 31 weeks all first-time mothers will be offered an antenatal check-up.

33–35 You will be offered an antenatal appointment at 34 weeks, and at least every 2 weeks from now on until your baby arrives. Expect to talk through your birth plan with your midwife or doctor by your 34-week appointment. See page 344 for help with your birth planning.

You may find it increasingly hard to tie your shoelaces, shave your legs or scramble around after a toddler as your bump gets in the way.

36 If this is your first pregnancy your baby may engage into your pelvis, preparing for birth, around now. You may notice that it's a bit easier to breathe and that you have less heartburn. The trade-off is a feeling of heaviness and pressure around your cervix and in your vagina. The classic late-pregnancy waddle often appears around now.

If your baby is breech at this point, you are likely to be offered an ECV (external cephalic version), to manually turn your baby by manipulating it from the outside. See page 242 for more information on breech babies.

If you haven't packed your birth bag yet, do it this week. Get your partner or birth partner to help you, so that they know what's in the bag and what it's for. Pack a bag even if you are planning a home birth, so that all the things you need are in one place and your partner doesn't present you with your honeymoon lingerie immediately after you've given birth.

Haemorrhoids can plague late pregnancy, particularly if this is your second or third time. Acupuncture can help, as well as traditional medicine, so don't suffer alone!

37

Congratulations, your baby is now considered to be ready to be born or 'full term'. It could well be weeks until you go into labour, though.

38

You'll probably be starting your maternity leave soon, if you haven't already.

Have you talked to close family and friends about your plans for visitors when you have a newborn? Setting boundaries that work for you is important, as is talking it through with your partner (more on page 352).

39 If you are having a planned caesarean it will likely happen around now. See page 195 for caesarean birth planning tips.

40 This is the week of your estimated due date (EDD) – estimated being the operative word. You only have a 4 per cent chance of having your baby on this date, so don't focus on it too much. Consider telling over-enthusiastic family that it's a week or two further on. Sixty per cent of you will have your baby a week either side of your due date, with 90 per cent giving birth within the 2 weeks either side.

41 If you are still pregnant beyond your due date, your midwife is likely to start talking about sweeps and offering you an induction of labour (often 9–12 days past your EDD). See page 247 for more information on these and alternatives to induction.

Nausea, some vomiting and diarrhoea can be a sign of impending labour. You might lose your mucus plug and feel increasingly crampy, achy and heavy too.

www.haveyouhadthatbabyyet.com is your new Facebook perma-status.

42

Because most women are induced before they reach 42 weeks there are very few pregnancies that continue past this point. Some women do choose to wait until their labour starts by itself – even past 42 weeks.

Chapter 2

Your Body

> " Anna: 'I loved my pregnant body. Much more than my usual one. I felt confident, my skin was great and I was proud of my belly.'
>
> Mariana: 'Urgh, pregnancy! That about sums it up. Apart from the lovely baby, the physical experience has nothing to recommend it. I just wanted to fast forward the whole 9 months and feel myself again.' "

Your body is important and there's no one it matters to more than you. Whether you feel positive about your physical self, or have had a more complicated relationship with the skin you live in, pregnancy can add a whole new dimension to your feelings.

There's an intense focus on your body during pregnancy, with you, your partner, family and friends, midwives, doctors and the world suddenly more interested in your diet, weight, exercise regime and health. Your body is changing by the day, with new sensations, symptoms and feelings to contend with all the time. It can be all tiny kicks, glossy hair, super-strong nails and neat little bump one minute and swollen-ankled, milk-leaking waddling the next.

And inside your body is another one – a whole new human growing within you. The responsibility of that can feel immense.

> **Mel: 'I have to confess I've never been a get fit, or "clean eating" kind of person. I've just bumbled along, taking my body for granted and not thinking about it too much – which has worked pretty well for me. But when I was pregnant I just found I cared about what I ate, actually enjoyed the yoga I'd signed up for. My body just made itself so obvious to me that I couldn't ignore it. I think being pregnant has actually made me feel more alive inside my body.'**

Almost all women gain weight during pregnancy, and this increase is so much more than just building fat stores. You gain another 50 per cent in blood volume, extra fluids, the placenta, amniotic fluid and the weight of your baby. And the fat stores you build are designed to take you through breastfeeding. It varies around the world, but in the UK there are no concrete guidelines on how much weight you should ideally gain in pregnancy. If you have a low BMI (body mass index) you'll be advised to try to gain more, and if you have a high BMI, guidance suggests you try to gain less. Australian information suggests a typical weight gain for someone with a normal-range BMI (18.5–24.9) might be between 11.3 and 15.9kg. But everyone is different, and this is a chance to listen to your body and work out what's right for you without getting too hung up on the numbers.

In this chapter I'll look at some of the body-related stuff that your pregnancy is likely to throw up. Pun intended. What you might choose to eat and drink, the decisions you'll make around exercise and how to decide what's right for you.

Whether your body is a temple of kale-filled purity, a shrine to the joys of the doughnut, or a more realistic combination of the two, I cross my heart and promise not to pester you with unachievable lists of things you must eat/do/avoid or drink. Instead I'll help you develop a realistic plan to help you feel as strong, healthy and ready for parenting as you can.

Your body matters because it's yours and it's got lots more work to do for you still. Don't let anyone convince you otherwise.

Your pregnancy body positive tips, by Danni, from the Chachi Power Project

1. Do not buy mainstream magazines. Turn the media dial right down now. Too much exposure to Photoshopped body types is not going to do you any favours. You look great – you got this.
2. Those stretch marks – every single one of them has a part to play in your little miracle. Remind yourself about that every time you see them.
3. Self-care is paramount. You MUST make sure that you are doing something nice for your mind or your body as much as possible. Of course checking into a spa is the dream, but how realistic is that? Spend as little as 30 seconds, once a day, if you can, focusing on you and how great you are. That could be a glance into the mirror to shout out loud, 'I am a fucking warrior,' or grabbing the hairbrush for a quick once-over on the barnet, or eating your fave bagel while leaning over the sink. Anything to recharge and have some 'me' time. This is a mental health must!

Preparing for pregnancy

If you're reading this before conception, hats off to you for forward planning. For some couples, taking control of their diet and exercise pre-conception can feel empowering, positive and a way to be even more actively involved in preparing to be parents. If this is you, or if you've been trying to conceive for over a year, then you may want to think about discussing your own and your partner's diet and exercise regimes (or lack of them!) with your GP or a specialist dietician. If you feel happy to carry on as you are, knowing that feeling relaxed and happy is also associated with fertility, then please do.

Perhaps the pre-conception phase has already passed and you are reading this over your expanding bump. If so, I want you to know that it's also OK not to prepare for pregnancy at all. Lots of us don't even intend to be pregnant and yet, there we are, 9 months later, holding a baby.

About 1 in 6 pregnancies is unplanned, and another nearly 30 per cent of pregnant women weren't actively trying to become pregnant when they conceived. And while that can be hard to hear for those who have had a long and bumpy road to conception, it's reassuring to know that, even if you don't prepare your body or bank account for a baby, you are going to do just fine. Don't panic if you didn't make any lifestyle changes prior to getting pregnant. Or if, like me, you spent the first 2 weeks of pregnancy unwittingly drinking bucket-sized gin and tonics.

Folic acid

Taking folic acid is the 'if you do one thing' recommendation for those of you trying to conceive, or who think you might be pregnant. Increased folic acid (vitamin B9) intake has been shown to help prevent neural tube defects, such as spina bifida, and may also play a part in helping reduce cleft lip and palate. The suggested dose for average women is a 400mcg supplement daily up until the end of the twelfth week of pregnancy – though it's safe to take throughout your pregnancy if you so wish. Diabetic women may be prescribed a higher dose. Folic acid is available over the counter, though you should be able to get a prescription if you need one.

Vitamin B9 naturally occurs as folate in green, leafy vegetables (kale again!), and folic acid is also an additive in some breakfast cereals and granary bread. There are theories that naturally occurring folate is more easily absorbed than folic acid supplements, but there's no reliable evidence to back up the protective effects of ditching the tablets and mainlining kale. Though as leafy vegetables have health benefits for you, there's certainly no harm in upping your natural folate intake too.

If you are unexpectedly pregnant and haven't been taking folic acid in advance or the early days, there's still no need to panic. There's only a very small chance of your baby developing a neural tube defect and your 20-week scan (see page 89) will be looking out for signs of any of these issues.

Eating in pregnancy

Advice on what and how much to eat is available in a range of often oh-so-helpfully conflicting formats. It also changes all the time. I was strongly warned against peanuts in my first pregnancy and actively encouraged to scoff them in my second. Myths abound, and it can be really hard to know what is 'safe' to eat when you are pregnant and to retain some perspective on just how important it is to follow the rules.

The only food rule I want to give you is to remember that your body will be prioritizing your baby's needs throughout your pregnancy. If you don't have a balanced and nutrient-rich diet you will divert any good stuff that is there to the baby, leaving you to function on almost nothing. If you focus on feeding yourself, fuelling your body for your life and ensuring that you are eating and drinking things to give you energy and resources, your baby will do just fine. Your body is taking care of your baby. Your job is to think about yourself.

Adele Hug is a registered dietician and I've asked her to cut through all the misinformation that's out there and put together some no-nonsense tips for you on what to eat and drink over the next 9 months.

'I spend most of my days dispelling food and nutrition myths – even sometimes to other health professionals,' says Adele. 'What works for one woman might not for another. You need to make it work for yourself and your partner/family. Every person is different and there isn't a one-food-fits-all approach.'

Adele's top 5 tips for thinking about diet and nutrition in your pregnancy

1. Balance!

- Try to eat a rainbow of about 5 different-coloured fruits and vegetables every day (fresh, tinned or frozen), for fibre, vitamins, polyphenols and antioxidants, to ensure you have all the nutrients you need to feel strong and well through pregnancy. By choosing lots of different colours and types you'll be getting a broad spectrum of nutrients without having to try too hard.

- Lean meats, pulses like lentils and beans, and vegetarian proteins (like soya and Quorn) will help support your muscles as they come under more strain.

- During pregnancy your body diverts calcium to your growing baby, but you still need some. Up your intake through dairy, or alternatives such as calcium-enriched nut milks, fish with bones, nuts and seeds.

- Pregnancy can make the most energetic of us desperate for a nap, so try to include some wholegrains (oats, brown rice, quinoa) and enjoy some more processed grains too (wholegrain bread, pasta) for energy and fibre.

- Nuts and seeds make a great protein-rich snack – try carrying some in your bag (along with other emergency nibbles) in case you get peckish while out and about.

- And don't forget about the good fats from foods like avocados, oily fish, and olive and rapeseed oils.

2. Food safety is more important than usual during pregnancy, as in some very rare cases specific foods or food preparation styles can lead to miscarriage, stillbirth or other problems. The official guidance on what food can pose particular risk can be found on the NHS website (www.nhs.uk/conditions/pregnancy-and-baby/pages/foods-to-avoid-pregnant.aspx). This guidance will currently warn you off eating raw, soft-boiled or poached eggs, but it's worth noting that this is likely to change soon, as research has shown that Lion kite-marked eggs in the UK present a very minimal risk of salmonella.

   Some women choose to follow the food rules to the letter during pregnancy, feeling safer and more confident knowing that they are avoiding anything that might increase their risk of a problem. Others, particularly those in their second or subsequent pregnancies, take each food on a case by case basis. You'll find your own way.

   Either way it's worth remembering that these food guidelines change reasonably frequently, with some 'unsafe' foods being declared safe and other safe foods being deemed problematic. If you accidentally eat a 'banned' food, remember that it may well be on the safe list in a few years' time.

3. Consider taking some supplements, but don't go overboard. If you have a truly balanced and rich diet (and

get plenty of sunlight), you might not bother. Otherwise pregnancy supplements should contain everything you need, but consider these specifics before deciding whether to supplement and, if so, what with:

- Vitamin D: All adults in the UK (including pregnant women) are encouraged to supplement at times when they aren't getting daily sun exposure on their bare skin. Adequate levels help keep your bones, teeth and muscles in tip-top shape. This vitamin occurs naturally in oily fish, eggs and red meat, so vegetarians and vegans may need to be particularly careful to get enough.

- Vitamin A: A balanced diet (perhaps including dairy, carrots, sweet potatoes and bloody kale again) should give you enough to boost your own immune system while your body diverts some to aid your baby's. Stay away from vitamin A supplements and foods high in vitamin A, like liver and liver pâté, as too much vitamin A can cause birth defects.

- Iodine: Supports your thyroid in regulating your hormones. Young women and pregnant women in the UK are prone to mild deficiency, so include some milk (especially non-organic milk) and white fish in your diet. Vegans may need to take an iodine supplement. See the Vegan Society for more information (www.vegansociety.com/sites/default/files/Iodine.pdf).

4. Trust yourself, listen to yourself and know when to ask for help. Try to stress less about food. There is and always will be well-meaning advice from us health professionals, friends, family and those pseudo-scientists out there. If you feel stressed by pregnancy food choices, ask your midwife for help.

Drinking alcohol

The official guidance on drinking alcohol in pregnancy has changed significantly over the past 15 years. The most recent guidance encourages women to abstain from alcohol entirely in pregnancy, citing evidence that persistent heavy drinking and binge-drinking can cause a range of problems for the growing foetus that can lead to foetal alcohol spectrum disorder (FASD).

Here's what the evidence base tells us:

- Babies of a small percentage of women who drink heavily in pregnancy (persistently, or in binges) will develop abnormally, leading to low IQ, facial deformity and a range of other complications. These are called foetal alcohol syndrome or foetal alcohol spectrum disorder.
- The chance of having complications is also related to the woman's wider health and socio-economic status, not just how much she drinks.
- Complications are hard to diagnose, but have life-long implications and can be on a spectrum from very serious to mild.

- There is no evidence that drinking small quantities of alcohol (such as 1–2 units once or twice a week) in pregnancy causes any harm at any stage.
- There have been some studies showing that moderate alcohol intake in pregnancy might lead to a greater chance of a lower birth-weight baby or an early baby.
- Some studies have shown that babies born to mothers who drink the equivalent of a glass of wine every day have no greater chance of foetal abnormalities. Some studies have found that low to moderate drinking increases the child's IQ.

It's important to know that:

- The Chief Medical Officer describes the advice to abstain from alcohol entirely as a 'precautionary' approach. Part of the rationale for this is that there isn't enough evidence of where the safe drinking limit is. There are also concerns that women may underestimate how much they are drinking, and that they might be drinking more units each week than they think.
- There is no evidence that drinking small amounts will harm your baby, but there is a belief that we need simple guidelines and that telling women not to drink anything is less likely to lead to confusion.
- There is no law on drinking in pregnancy and no one can or should refuse to serve you or sell you alcohol in pregnancy.
- If you drank alcohol before finding out you were pregnant, don't worry. Unless you discovered your

pregnancy much later than normal (in which case it's worth having a frank chat with your midwife or doctor, who will likely be very reassuring), this is incredibly common and there is no evidence that it will have any impact on your baby.

Making your own drinking decision

My approach was to steer clear in the first trimester – I just didn't feel like it. I had a couple of glasses of wine in the later weeks of my first pregnancy and one or two small drinks a week in my second.

> Claire : 'I didn't much fancy knocking back a beer when I was feeling nauseous but by about 18 weeks I did sometimes crave one. I looked it up and discovered there wasn't actually any reason why I couldn't have the occasional beer, so I did! It was lovely. I did get a few funny looks when I ordered half a pint on a night out, so I made sure to pat my bump particularly visibly when I did as a way of helping them mind their own business.'
>
> Kate: 'I had both my babies when you were told it was OK to drink a little bit, but I couldn't understand why anyone would risk it. I didn't want to eat or drink anything that had even the tiniest chance of harming my baby, and the thought of doing so would have made me feel awful. I took a tour of juices and soft drinks and discovered that you can convince yourself that your gin-less tonic tastes exactly the same as the real deal.'

By looking at the guidelines and evidence for yourself and listening to your instincts, you can make a decision on what's right for you.

Eating disorders in pregnancy

Around 670,000 women in the UK have an eating disorder. If you have recovered from an eating disorder or have one at the moment, it's very common for previous patterns of eating to re-emerge in pregnancy.

For some women with an eating disorder, pregnancy actually helps aid recovery and helps them control their symptoms. Whatever your reaction, it's important to ensure you get the right emotional and practical support through your pregnancy. Tell your midwife about your current or previous experiences, symptoms and treatment. If you need support to ensure that you can eat the kind of food in enough volume to meet your own and your baby's basic needs, your midwife and GP can refer you to a dietician or specialist therapist and should offer you support from the perinatal mental health team.

Polly, who had severe anorexia and depression in her teens and early twenties, had recovered by the time she became pregnant at 24.

 'I wasn't sure if was able to have kids – my periods still hadn't returned after stopping when I was ill. But my partner and I wanted to take any chance we had, so we didn't do anything to prevent me getting pregnant in the hope it may happen some day. Eventually out of the blue it did! I

found out by accident, as I had to take a test
before an X-ray and it was positive! I loved my
bump and changing body, but I know many
women struggle with this.'

"

Polly finds listening to body positive podcasts such as
Fearless Rebelle Radio, Food Psych and The Love, Food Podcast
helps her with her relationship with food and her body.

Exercise

Pregnancy is probably not the logical time to start running marathons, hang-gliding or base jumping if your regime to date has comprised a gentle stroll to the remote and back. Nor is it any reason to abandon the activity you love. As with diet, doing what works for you, getting risks and benefits into perspective and focusing on what is going to make you feel good in your changing body is the way forward.

As a guideline:

- Don't start a very hardcore new exercise regime, but feel free to carry on with the exercise you like. Do tell your instructor or trainer about your pregnancy as soon as you find out. You may need to gradually dial it down as you become less mobile and your lung capacity decreases.
- If you are keen to stay fit and active you might find the exercises available at Mumhood by Frame perfect throughout pregnancy and after: www.mum-hood.com.

- If you haven't exercised much to date, you can still enjoy walking, swimming and pregnancy-specific exercise such as aqua-natal and pregnancy yoga classes. If you have specific health concerns or mobility issues, check in with your medical team and the class instructor first.
- If you are doing something with significant danger attached (horse riding, skiing, mountain climbing), do a realistic risk assessment and think about how safe it feels to you, now you are pregnant.

Should you exercise? I'm not one to tell you what to do, but I secretly think it might be a good idea. Not for aesthetic reasons, but because many women find it hard to find time to focus on themselves even before the demands of mother-hood are clawing at their diary. Doing things to nurture our bodies and minds (rather than improve them) is not something we've often been encouraged to do. In the pressurized world we live in it's vital to make space for looking after our bodies and minds in pregnancy and to set up good habits for motherhood.

We are also often not accustomed to really understanding, consciously inhabiting and thinking about our bodies and connecting with them. In pregnancy, when so much is happening inside our bodies and with the prospect of childbirth on the horizon, it can be useful to get back in touch with the skin we are in.

With that in mind, I'll encourage you to give some pregnancy yoga a try, as it can help calm the mind, strengthen the body and help you get the two a little more in synch. You can find a class local to you, or work through some of the books and DVDs suggested on the resources website.

To get you in the mood, I've included a simple yoga breathing practice in each part of the book, put together by yoga expert Ashley Macdonald. I'm presuming you are already pretty gifted at breathing – it's been keeping you successfully alive for some time. But doing some regular yoga-inspired breathing work can help you feel calmer, lessen insomnia and encourage you to tune in to how your body and mind might work together. It'll give you a headstart for the labour breathing practice on page 174, too.

Breathing practice 1: Moving breath

You can do this breathing at any time of day – though before bed is good for insomniacs. Find a place to sit comfortably and quietly if you have one, ideally cross-legged if that's comfortable for you. On the tube or at your desk could also work as long as you aren't a heavy breather.

- Place your relaxed hands on your abdomen. Inhale, trying to breathe the air directly into the place your hands are resting on. Feel your hands move away from each other and away from your spine. As you exhale, feel them hug back into one another. Do this 5 more times, concentrating on focusing your breath a little more each time into the place where your hands are.

- Then move your hands up to between your bra-line and the bottom of your ribs. Your thumbs will be round the back of your rib cage and your fingers fanned out around the front. Breathe into the place where your hands are now. Feel your hands being pushed away from the centre of your body as you inhale, and when you exhale, feel them fan back inwards. Do this 5 more times, concentrating on isolating your breath a little more each time into the place where your hands are.

- Now move your hands up to your collarbone, placing the fingers of your right hand on the right side of your collarbone and those of your left hand on the other. Now breathe into this much higher place. You'll feel your collarbone rising as you breathe in and sinking back down as you breathe out. Notice how you feel as you do this 5 more times.

- It's hard to isolate these different places to breathe, even with lots of practice, so be patient and kind to yourself.

- Once you've tried these separately, it's time to put them together. In one inhalation, breathe first into your belly, then your ribs and then your collarbone. You can move your hands, not use them, or have one lower and one higher – whatever works for you. When you exhale, do so first from your collarbone, then your ribs and then your belly. Do this 5 more times.

- Before you open your eyes and finish, do 3 normal breaths.

High BMI

Two in 10 pregnant women in the UK have a BMI of over 30. It is pretty common, and while there are certainly some particular risks that are elevated, these need to be looked at in a proportionate and non-sensational way. However, recent surveys and studies have shown that many women with a high BMI feel their care focuses too much on the risks, and isn't sensitive or helpful.

If you want to get to grips with the reality rather than the hype, there's good support out there if you know where to look. The Big Birthas website (www.bigbirthas.co.uk) is run by Amber Marshall, whose own pregnancy and birth experiences with a high BMI led her to collect together the evidence, along with women's stories, to give a more realistic picture. She explains that many women she has spoken to mistakenly believe that they're almost guaranteed to have problems of one sort or another due to their size – and are surprised to hear that the odds are on their side when it comes to having a normal, unproblematic birth.

If you have a higher BMI you are likely to be offered support from a specialist clinic during your pregnancy and will be referred there by your midwife. You might find this a really helpful source of information, as they are often run by highly expert midwives or obstetricians with some relevant services for you, your pregnancy and your baby. But it is worth remembering that, however this referral is presented to you, it is not mandatory and you do not have to attend if you don't want to.

Diabetes

If you are diagnosed with gestational diabetes in pregnancy, or already have type 1 or type 2 diabetes, speak to your maternity team for a referral to a specialist registered dietician. Adele's advice is to find one you can be honest and open with and whose advice you trust.

Checklist

1. Notice what you love about your pregnancy body and give yourself time to get used to what you aren't so keen on. See the body positive tips on page 22.
2. Are you taking folic acid yet? (See page 24.)

3. Understand the guidelines for eating and drinking in pregnancy and make your own decision about what's right for you (see page 25).
4. Read pages 33–5 on exercise in pregnancy and make your personal exercise plan (see page 340).
5. Have you tried the 'moving breath' yoga practice yet? (See page 35.)

Chapter 3

Your Mind

> **❝** 'We alter enormously in pregnancy. Our brains undergo changes similar to those of our teenage years – seeing a reduction in grey matter (making it more concentrated), and the rapid formation of new connections. We also see an increase in activity in the amygdala – our brain's alarm system. This makes us hypersensitive to our child's needs but also explains why we may find ourselves feeling more anxious than expected. Hormonally, during pregnancy and early motherhood we have a huge increase in oxytocin, which can improve our social skills, increase our sensitivity to others and ease stress. If we can embrace these changes and see them as an opportunity for learning and growth, they can feel very positive.'
> – Emma Svanberg, clinical psychologist **❞**

If you only have time to read one chapter of this book, let it be this one. The care you get, the books you read and the focus of those around you can make you think that preparing for motherhood is all about your body and getting it to behave. Thinking about the physical, in an empowering way, is important, but it's far from being all there is to it. Working

40

out how you are going to emerge at the end of this incredible 9-month journey feeling as mentally well and robust as possible needs to take pride of place in your plans.

The demands of parenting can be massive. And though the rewards are also huge, you will need support, acknowledgement, practical information and tools to help you strike out into motherhood feeling good about yourself and ready for this next phase of your life, in which someone else will be relying on you for emotional support. The evidence is pretty clear – many women face mental ill-health issues in pregnancy. These aren't spoken about enough, leading to people feeling frightened or ashamed and not seeking support. Women's mental health and wellbeing during pregnancy, birth and parenting has been hiding up in the attic, getting gradually dustier, moth-eaten and more fragile, while a focus on getting things right for our bodies has become an obsession downstairs.

Thankfully there's now growing awareness that lots of women find the transition to motherhood difficult and that looking after our minds as well as our vaginas is probably a good idea. It's just that we aren't used to doing it yet. Let's change that! Your mind matters. It matters because it is what makes you you, and, as you should know by now, you are of utmost importance.

Most of us, myself included, don't spend much time thinking in advance about the impact of pregnancy and parenthood on our emotions, our brains, our sense of self or our relationships with those around us. But becoming a parent can lift the lid on a host of strange, wonderful and difficult feelings about ourselves. Being prepared and getting a handle on how you feel before your time is filled with daily baby wrangling is a really good idea.

How pregnancy might make you feel

" Lia: 'Like me – only rounder.'

Preeti: 'I felt like I was on this fast-moving train and even though I didn't want to get off, something about the fact I couldn't made me feel anxious and doubt myself.'

Millie: 'Wonderful! Sure, I had my crying-at-loo-roll-ads moments of madness, but I basically felt fan-fucking-tastic as soon as the pukey phase ended.' **"**

Only you can know how your pregnancy will make you feel. And it can change wildly across those 9 months and from one pregnancy to the next. The phrase 'anything goes' has never been so appropriate, and the spectrum really does go from feelings of joy and connection with the world to dark and deep depression and everything in between.

However you feel is OK – unless it doesn't feel OK for you. Some women love pregnancy, connect instantly with their growing baby, look forward to motherhood and find the rest of life an annoying distraction.

But, as Phoebe found, you might feel distant from the pregnancy:

" 'I felt a bit like I was going through the motions. Everyone wanted to talk about it but, for me, it wasn't real until I was holding the baby and even then it took a while. I feel sad now that I felt like I had to perform this role of hyper-excited mother-to-be when actually I was just the same old me.' **"**

Relationships with others

" Teresa: 'Becoming parents together has made
my boyfriend and I closer, more connected
and our relationship is deeper. We understand
each other more and have this massive
experience in common.'

Michelle: 'There were some moments when I
thought we might not get through this without
breaking up. We are, but it has taken more work
than I imagined and I wish, wish, wish we'd
been better prepared.' **"**

Pregnancy presents a range of emotional and relationship-
based challenges and opportunities. One of the biggest
can be the impact on how you feel about your friends, parents, family and partner – as well as how they feel about and
treat you.

As parent/child psychotherapist Kitty Hagenbach explains,
'Children download family dynamics without any filter and
family issues remain in our unconscious. Being pregnant and
having a baby often brings these hidden dynamics to our
consciousness.'

Looking ahead to turning into parents ourselves can lead
us suddenly and unexpectedly to reconsider the way we were
parented. As our parents also move up the chain towards
grandparenting, all sorts of long-forgotten emotions can come
to the surface. It can be a chance to work things through,
improve relationships and set off towards parenting on the
best foot.

> Suzi: 'I just suddenly had an insight into what it meant to be a parent and I felt so grateful to my mum for going through it all for me. We had more open conversations than ever before and I suddenly felt like we were equals.'

> Anya: 'I hadn't spoken to my mother for five years. Being pregnant I just found myself re-hashing it all in my head. I did think about getting back in touch but decided to go back to a therapist I'd worked with before to work through it. Through that I realized I needed to focus on my new family for now. It really shocked me, though, how I plunged back into all that stuff and I did really need my partner and the professionals to get me through it.'

It can also be a hard time if you have a parent missing from your life. Linda's mother died when she was 15; she remembers feeling lonely in pregnancy and grieving for her all over again. Grief support can help, even if your parent died a long time ago. Try Cruse Bereavement Care (0808 808 1677 or www.cruse.org.uk) as your first port of call.

Other relationships can go through changes in pregnancy, most importantly the one with your partner. As each of you goes on your own subconscious journey, thinking about how you were parented and working out what kind of parent you want to be, it can be a real chance for open discussions that set a good foundation for the months and years ahead.

> Fran: 'After a rough IVF journey we started the pregnancy having forgotten why we were doing this, but the whole thing just helped heal what

we'd been through. We started being more open
and loving again. Evie was totally blown away
by how I was coping with it all and I felt like we
were more connected than ever.'

Angela: 'We were both so excited when we found
out I was pregnant but Mark became less and less
interested, was at work longer hours and we were
sniping at each other. We had a massive row and I
said something awful to him about the baby being
better off without a dad like him and then it all kind
of clicked for both of us. He didn't know his dad,
who'd left when his mum was pregnant and,
without realizing, he'd started feeling depressed
about all of that and wasn't able to connect with
what was happening now. Just acknowledging and
talking to each other helped instantly.'

**Emma Svanberg's plan for
becoming parents – together**

1. Spend some time reflecting on your personality, and how
   that might influence your parenting. Do you like to feel in
   control of things? Or are you more of a free spirit? How
   do you react when plans change – do you find it stressful
   or not? This can help you when it comes to making
   decisions about your parenting later on – there's no point
   in doing what your hippy best friend is doing if routine is
   all important to you, that's a path to misery.

2. Reflect on your experiences as a child. What were your parents like? What parts of their parenting would you like to replicate? And which bits do you now feel you'd like to do differently? Discuss this with your partner too.
3. Talk at length with your partner about how you want to protect your relationship – and keep talking after the baby is born. You are suddenly not the most important person in the world to each other and that can take some negotiating.
4. Start to notice how you deal with anxiety and stress in your day-to-day life. Don't be afraid to ask for help with anxiety management strategies. See page 171 for ideas.

Tension release exercise

Feeling stressed? This exercise can be a quick and easy way to notice tension, release it and calm your mind. If you practise it in pregnancy it will also be really useful in your labour. However, if you've experienced sexual violence or physical trauma, this exercise might be triggering. Instead, try adapting the fear release exercise on page 171 to help you let go of any worries and tension.

Be comfortable sitting or lying down. In the bath can work too. Close your eyes and breathe normally, in through your nose and out through your mouth. When your breathing is relaxed and slow, imagine, as you breathe in through your nose, that the air goes straight into the top of your head and across your scalp. Take several breaths into that place and notice any tension, tightness or pain in that part of your body. Then, as you breathe out through your mouth, feel that tension leaving the top of your head with your out breath. Do several breath cycles until this part of your body feels supple, strong and light.

Make your way gradually down your body, one area at a time. You might want to include:

- Your face

- The back of your neck

- Your shoulders

- Down your arms into your fingers, the tips of which may tingle as you exhale

- Your ribcage and lungs

- Your upper back

- All the way down your spine

- Your lower back and hips

- Your abdomen, where your baby is

- Your pelvis, also cradling your baby

- Your bottom and thighs

- Your knees and down your shins and calves

- Your ankles and feet

- Your toes, which may also tingle as you exhale

When you've worked through your body, do 5 breaths going from head to toe to catch any areas you've missed. Before you open your eyes, notice how your body and then your mind is feeling. If you notice you store tension in one or two areas of your body every time, you can do a quick-fire relax of just these areas if you need to feel calmer in a hurry.

Common mental health issues in pregnancy

As you'll know by now, it's normal for pregnancy to make you feel emotionally different. Happily most women don't experience mental ill-health in pregnancy, but it is more common than many of us realize. If you've had previous mental health issues, you might find that pregnancy triggers them once again. If you have ongoing mental health issues, pregnancy could change, worsen or relieve your symptoms. But even if you've had a clean bill of mental health in the past, you might find that pregnancy brings a mental health condition to light or triggers something new.

Dr Rebecca Moore explains that mental health changes in pregnancy are quite common. 'One in seven women have some mood change during pregnancy but half of them don't seek help. If you are struggling please tell someone how you are feeling. Help is available and with support you will feel better.'

If you have a pre-existing mental illness, do consider telling your midwife about this at your booking appointment or the next early opportunity. 'Don't be afraid or ashamed,' says Dr Moore. 'The more aware the team are, the more they can support you.' Mental health issues are so common that most areas routinely ask a series of standardized screening questions to look for past and current mental health issues during the booking appointment.

Medication

If you are currently taking medication to help you control a mental illness, you don't need to suddenly stop it in pregnancy, as this could trigger a relapse. Instead see your GP and/or specialist as soon as you know that you are pregnant. They should be able to help you weigh up the risks and benefits of stopping or continuing your medication and suggest suitable alternatives if appropriate.

If you develop a pregnancy-related mental health condition, or are struggling with feelings of depression, anxiety or compulsion, remember that medication isn't always necessary. As Dr Moore explains, 'There are often a range of options available aside from medication and many milder cases can be treated with diet, exercise and therapy.'

Antenatal depression

Though postnatal depression gets all the headlines, 1 in 10 pregnant women will experience depression that starts in pregnancy, not after birth. You might feel low all the time, constantly tired, unable to enjoy life, sad, tearful, irritable, have altered sleep patterns, a changed appetite and lack of concentration. Sometimes women may feel more on edge and worried – especially about their health or the pregnancy.

Of course some of these symptoms are part and parcel of a normal pregnancy, but if you feel something is up, are finding it hard to cope or can't function in your usual way, you might be suffering from antenatal depression and it's time to seek help from your doctor or midwife.

Some women have delayed seeking help because of fear that a diagnosis of depression might mean their baby is at risk of being taken away. Dr Moore has worked in this field for nearly 20 years and has 'never seen a baby removed from a mother solely due to depression. Feeling low or anxious in pregnancy does not make you a bad person or a bad mum. Depression is very treatable and the prognosis is very good. We are not there to judge or criticize and want to support you back to health.'

Other issues

Anxiety is another common issue that can come up in pregnancy. If you are feeling worried and tense all the time, particularly anxious about birth or being a good enough mother, it's worth seeking some support.

Obsessive Compulsive Disorder (OCD) can occur or re-occur in pregnancy too. Some women find they are plagued by recurrent intrusive thoughts or images. This can lead to associated repetitive behaviours that can make it difficult to go about their day-to-day life. Angela became increasingly fearful about germs during her pregnancy. 'It was like I could actually see them on everything around me. People's hands, my house, the car, my keyboard at work. It started off with using hand sanitizer and wiping things, but soon escalated out of control and I really couldn't work any more, or go to friends' houses. Public transport was completely impossible.'

The treatment plans for these conditions will be tailored to you and will also depend on what's available in your area. For Angela, recovery took a while but she did get better: 'My mother eventually made me go and talk to my GP, who was really switched on to OCD and got me referred straight away. I had cognitive behavioural therapy (CBT), which is a kind of talking therapy that helps rewire your brain not to go down the compulsive behaviour route. If it hadn't worked so well I could have had drugs as well, but I didn't need them. I did find I had a bit of a relapse after the baby was born, but I knew how to get help this time and so I managed to get on top of it quickly.'

Tocophobia

As many as 1 in 10 pregnant women suffer with a severe fear of childbirth called tocophobia. It's very normal to feel anxious or stressed by the thought of giving birth – especially if you haven't done it before.

But for some women their feelings about birth go well beyond this. If you think you might be one of them, your midwife should be able to discuss your concerns, offer reassurance and help you feel more confident. Information is often key to relieving anxiety, so get yourself clued up on your options, read other women's stories and check out the range of support groups such as the brilliant Positive Birth Movement (www.positivebirthmovement.org).

Dr Moore's advice is that if the anxiety is severe and more persistent, CBT or brief psychotherapy could be really helpful. For some women, fear of childbirth might be connected to something traumatic from their past. If you have suffered childhood sexual abuse, sexual violence, a traumatic accident or injury or have post-traumatic stress disorder, you might find that these experiences and any trauma symptoms impact on how you feel about giving birth. In Chapter 12 there are a range of exercises and suggestions for women who've had a previously traumatic birth, and you may find these really helpful for you, even if the trauma you've had wasn't directly related to childbirth.

On www.rebeccaschiller.co.uk/noguilt you'll find some specific books, support groups and suggestions for trauma survivors and survivors of sexual abuse or violence. It can be really difficult to open up to your midwife about trauma or sexual violence in your past, but if you feel able to – at any point during your pregnancy – then it should enable your team to minimize the situations, procedures and phrases that might trigger you.

Checklist

1. Think about how pregnancy is making you feel. How can you turn the dial up on the positive and get help with the negative? (See page 42.)
2. Talk through your experiences of being parented and your hopes for how you will parent with your partner (see page 43).
3. Practise the tension release exercise (see page 46) at least once a week. Notice where you hold tension – it will be useful in labour (see page 176).
4. Talk through any pre-existing mental health issues and make a plan with your midwife or doctor (see page 48).

Chapter 4

Your Life

> ❝ Callie: 'Look at my face, not my uterus! Gah, it drives me bonkers how once you are pregnant everyone assumes you are just a walking incubator. I love being pregnant but I still love other stuff too.' ❞

You might be pregnant but, shock horror, you still have a life. Sure, it's changing rapidly and shifting around to accommodate another person, but you remain completely, 100 per cent, you. You are still allowed to care about your work, your friendships, your bank balance and your career.

For many of us, pregnancy and impending motherhood impacts on our lives outside of the baby bubble in much bigger, better and more confusing ways than traditional pregnancy preparation gives us space to acknowledge.

You are more than your pregnancy, so in this chapter I'll focus on how it bumps up against the rest of your life.

Work

For the majority of pregnant women, reconciling pregnancy and parenthood with work life is a necessity that's hard to do. Thankfully, employees in the UK have rights to paid time off for antenatal appointments, flexibility about when to start maternity leave, a good chunk of paid time off after the baby is born, opportunities to share that with their partner, and protection of their job while they are off work. It's a trickier picture if you are self-employed or do casual or agency work.

I'll set out some of these rights here, and will also point you to where you can get more detailed information and support. Knowledge is power, so make sure you know what you are entitled to in case your employer does not.

Telling work

You need to tell your employer about your pregnancy by week 25. You may want to tell them much earlier and, if you are anything like me (who swells up like Michelin Man's heftier sister), they may guess well before. If you are self-employed it's up to you if and when you tell your clients and others you may work with.

The amount and type of maternity leave and pay you are entitled to will depend on whether you are employed or self-employed, whether you became pregnant before or after you started your job, how much you earn and whether your company has any additional maternity benefits. Confusing? It certainly is. But fear not, Maternity Action has detailed factsheets covering almost all circumstances and eventualities, so use them to get clued up. You'll find their factsheets and telephone advice line number on their website, www.maternityaction.org.uk.

Maternity leave

> **Cait: 'In pregnancy I was desperate to have the baby and get back to work as quickly as possible. After the baby was here I realized I did need some time to recover and get my body and brain back on track. I went back at 10 months which was just about perfect.'**
>
> **Lisa: 'I was freelancing again by week 6 and working as much as usual by the time she was 4 months old. I loved it and I needed to do it for money and my sanity.'**
>
> **Yessica: 'She was born and in that moment I knew I was never going to go back to my old job. I will work again, but not until they are in school. And parenting is work – hard work at that!'**

In the UK, employees must take the first 2 weeks off after childbirth. If you work in a factory, be prepared for that minimum leave period to increase to 4 weeks.

Many of you will be entitled to 26 weeks of ordinary maternity leave (OML), after which your employer must ensure that you can return to exactly the same job if you want to. You might choose to take some or all of your additional maternity leave (AML), which lasts for another 26 weeks.

As I know only too well, if you are self-employed it can be much harder to plan a maternity leave. Those of us running our own business often find it hard to set aside a small window of time for totally switching off from work. I confess to taking work calls in the first week of life with my second baby, though I did so from bed, topless, breastfeeding while my toddler sprinkled toast crumbs on the sheets.

If you are a casual or agency worker I'm afraid you don't qualify for any maternity leave unless it states so in your contract, but all is not lost – you may still be able to get pay through a 'Maternity Allowance' (see www.gov.uk/maternity-allowance).

Maternity pay

To make things as confusing as possible, maternity leave and maternity pay are two entirely different things that operate in a mysterious, overlapping Venn diagram kind of way. You may qualify for one but not the other, and the amount of time for which you will be entitled to leave is unlikely to match the length of time for which you are entitled to pay. Luckily for those of us who need to figure out what we're entitled to, baby brain has been shown to be a myth.

You can get up-to-date information about what maternity leave and pay you are entitled to on the Maternity Action website (www.maternityaction.org.uk).

If you need or want to keep one foot in the door of work, check in with your team, or keep your contacts and contracts from disappearing elsewhere if you are self-employed, then it's good to know that you can take up to 10 'keeping in touch' (KIT) days to do your normal work without losing entitlement to your leave or pay.

Don't forget about paternity leave

Depending on how long they've been employed, your partner may be able to claim up to 2 weeks' paid paternity leave after the baby is born. If you have a female partner, are not married or your partner (who is going to have some responsibility for caring for the child) is not the child's father, they will still be able to claim paternity leave if they meet the employment criteria.

This leave needs to be taken in a single chunk and needs to be used within 56 days (who picks these random numbers?!) of your baby's birth.

Shared parental leave

> **Alice: 'Ben works part-time so I can work in an office for a few days a week knowing the kids are all sorted. In fact it is one of my favourite things to come home after a hard day at the office to find the house tidy, a hot meal on the table and the kids in the bath and all sorted! Lush!'**

Thankfully it's now – at least theoretically – acknowledged that just because we are the pregnant ones doesn't mean that those of us who happen to have uteruses make better stay-at-home parents. Happily there's much more than paternity leave on the table, and shared parental leave gives employees and their partners a chance to flex and share maternity leave. When it works, it can enable women to return to work earlier without having to rely on traditional or paid-for childcare.

Alice and Ben were one of the first couples to try out shared leave in 2015 after the birth of their third child, Ada. 'We thought it was time to be more equal and for Ben to have a go. Plus three young children is hard work – having Ben working full-time at the same time would have been almost impossible. Ben's employer was pretty supportive but he was trailblazing – he had to work closely with HR to come up with a plan. He's still seen as a little strange for doing it and no one has followed him since.'

All three of the couple's babies were initially breastfed, then mixed fed. Since Alice worked from home she was able to breastfeed when need be, although the couple think Ada probably did get more bottles and breastfed a bit less than her siblings, as she was with her dad much more.

Alice and Ben took the first 3 weeks of leave off together. Alice then took her leave before swapping with Ben when Ada was 4 months old.

Alice and Ben think it is 'so important for all men to take as much parental leave as they possibly can, partly so they get what it's like (not easy!) but also so they get that invaluable chance to bond with their children'.

Work problems and challenges

The first few months of pregnancy can often be the most challenging for those of us juggling work and the contents of our uterus: unparalleled exhaustion, weird mood swings, feeling nauseous (or actually being sick) at a time when we are often trying to keep the news on a need-to-know basis. Consider telling your boss sooner rather than later, so that they can help you come up with a work plan that is sympathetic to your early pregnancy symptoms. Working from home to avoid nausea-inducing public transport, changing your hours and resting at lunchtime might help. Your employer should also ensure that they've done a health and safety assessment for you, especially if you have a physical or dangerous job.

Most employers will be keen to support you and make

sure you get what you are entitled to. If you are having prob-lems getting your employer to do the right thing by your maternity rights, Joeli Brearley, founder of Pregnant Then Screwed, has some tips for you.

'The first thing to do is talk to your employer. Often issues can be solved with very open communication. If that doesn't work then start writing everything down in detail, logging every episode. You should also ensure things that are said to you are confirmed in writing. Call Acas immediately and then call Pregnant Then Screwed's free legal advice line on 0161 930 5300 or email on advice@pregnantthenscrewed.com and we will be able to tell you where you stand and can support you through the whole process from that point forwards.'

Sex

> Emma: 'In my first pregnancy I felt constantly horny in the second trimester and had some great sex with my female partner. But I found catching sight of my belly, or feeling the baby kick, massively off-putting and worried my partner did too. After a few miscarriages in between I felt much more worried about orgasms in my second pregnancy. I had an irrational fear that it would shake the baby out in the first trimester and avoided sex a bit, which is unusual for me.'

We've already thought about how pregnancy might impact on your relationships, and with another future person in the mix you'll definitely find it has some impact on your sex life. Will your libido reach hitherto unimagined levels that exceed even the wettest of dreams? Or will you shut up the orgasm shop for a few months? I'll hold my hands up and say I don't know and neither will anyone else, but most women find their normal sex drive alters during their pregnancy. One study (see www.rebeccaschiller.co.uk/noguilt) found that although the amount of sex women were having generally decreased during their pregnancies, satisfaction and desire were relatively unchanged throughout. Most women in the study (75 per cent) didn't experience any specific sexual problems. Those who did find sex tricky talked about pain during penetration, difficulty reaching orgasm, lack of vaginal lubrication and low desire.

Cherry, Anniki and Lisa from the Hotbed Collective:

'Pregnancy can give you bigger, more sensitive boobs which are a great starting point for sexy play. The swelling stomach and idea that your body is a sacred space during pregnancy help many women feel body confident, focusing on the positives of their physicality rather than any perceived inadequacies. The hormone oxytocin surges throughout pregnancy, giving many women an increased appetite for sex, masturbation and experimentation.'

If you aren't feeling it, Caroline, who is part of The Good Sex (a project that explores and supports the relationship between women today and sexuality), thinks that the biggest myth around being pregnant and sexuality is the idea that every pregnant woman suddenly has a surge in sexual desire:

'I've had women look to me for reassurance that it is normal also to not want sex during pregnancy. This has been my personal experience and I think it's one that's overlooked. As a result it leads to women feeling guilty and isolated as they think they're not "normal" because their libido is lower.'

> Paula: 'The idea of sex makes me cringe. All the wobble, the awkwardness. I miss sex and love my husband but I have no desire to jump on him.'

> Yemi: 'The more pregnant I was, the more I felt like sex, which was tricky as I didn't have a partner. It became a bit of an overwhelming compulsion and I did masturbate a lot. I did go on a couple of dates with open-minded women but, though I was really into the idea of having sex, I felt too weird about something casual when I was pregnant.'

Dr Karen Gurney (a clinical psychologist specializing in sexual problems) explains that sexual issues are quite common in pregnancy and that it's helpful for you and your partner to be aware of this and know that these changes are likely to be transitory and related to the effects of pregnancy, childbirth, being a new parent or breastfeeding, not related to a problem within the couple. Nausea might be a turn-off in the first trimester and tiredness in the third, but Karen suggests trying to maintain as much of a physical relationship as you can. If penetrative sex becomes uncomfortable, continue to have other types of sex such as oral sex. If sexual contact feels too difficult altogether, she recommends prioritizing other types of physical intimacy so that you and your partner find other ways to make each other feel attractive and wanted.

You don't need me to tell you that sex isn't going to bash the baby, but partners sometimes need reassurance. If you feel like having sex, you might have to experiment with different positions towards the end of your pregnancy to work out what's comfortable for you.

> ❝ Rosie: 'For us it was definitely no missionary position after 20 weeks because my bump was too big. He's a very petite man and I would just feel too whale-like to be on top, so that's out too. We've found a side-by-side scissoring position to be the only one that works now, with my husband touching me at the same time.' ❞

It's normal for sex, and orgasm in particular, to trigger Braxton Hicks contractions. Sex is one of the classic home-induction techniques and, with a combination of prostaglandins in semen, orgasm stimulating the uterus to contract and oxytocin levels heightening, it makes sense. But fear not, sex will only trigger a labour that's absolutely about to start anyway. You only need to avoid it in pregnancy if your midwife or doctor has advised you against it or if your waters have broken.

If you aren't feeling like having sex – don't! It's up to you.

Money

> ❝ Lucy: 'I was saving up for my maternity leave during pregnancy. Squirrelling away as much as I possibly could so that, as the highest earner, I could stay off for longer with my baby. I googled "thrifty pregnancy" about 100 times, begged and borrowed

almost everything I needed. I didn't want to feel like
my partner was giving me an allowance while I was
on maternity leave and I still wanted to be able to
buy myself the odd treat without feeling like I
was frittering away his hard-earned money.' **"**

Having a baby makes most of us think hard about money
and wish we had more. From what to buy and how to budget
for it, to saving for maternity leave, adjusting to earning less,
or being more reliant on your partner's income as well as
what you can and want to spend on your pregnancy and
birth – money is definitely an object.

I know that going from being the higher earner to greatly
reduced maternity pay and then earning nothing felt like it
rocked my identity. Do some planning and talking with your
partner, so that changes to your bank balance and your
financial relationship with each other don't come as a shock.

Coping with financial changes

Babies mean more expense at a time when most of us are
earning less. Get ahead of the game and start planning for
money changes now.

1. Do a financial audit of your and your partner's weekly
   spending to see where the money goes.
2. Agree on a new budget during your pregnancy, ideally
   setting aside some savings to use when your salary drops.
3. Discuss your approach to sharing (or not) your earnings
   when you are on leave. Who will pay for baby-related

If you buy baby magazines, switch on the TV or visit Instagram you may well think that babies need a huge amount of very expensive kit. Making one baby-related purchase can lead you down an advertising wormhole that can leave even the most sensible of us wondering if we need to sell an organ to have a child. I call bullshit on this. Many pregnancies are not planned. Some of us haven't been saving for years to provide a nest egg for our maternity leave and the things we need to buy. Contrary to what we are led to believe, babies have pretty simple, inexpensive needs. When I was Anna's doula, she went into labour at 37 weeks, before they had bought a single thing for the baby. Her husband, Paul, went to the shops while I took her home where she had the baby a few hours later. His small carrier bag full of vests, nappies and a couple of other bits and bobs was supplemented by presents from friends. Some parenting choices later (no buggy and no cot), and they estimated that they spent £800 in total in the first year compared with the whopping £5,200 parents spend on average. A baby on a budget can be done.

Baby shopping essentials

1. **Somewhere for your baby to sleep:** There are lots of options, from moses baskets to cribs and cots.

Borrowing a second-hand moses basket for the first few months and then purchasing a second-hand cot, or an inexpensive new one (try Ikea for cheap and functional cots), is probably the cheapest solution for sleeping separately to your baby. Co-sleeping (when babies share their mother's beds) requires no equipment, but do read the safety information on page 278.

2. **A way to transport your baby:** A car seat is a must unless you will never be in a car with your newborn. Prams/buggies can be big bucks, so look on eBay and ask friends for bargains. Slings and baby carriers are cheaper than a buggy, so if you think you may want to babywear, start by attending a local sling meeting to try different styles out. Some people avoid the expense of a buggy by exclusively babywearing at least at first, until cheaper buggies for older babies become an option.

3. **Baby clothes (but not too many) and some muslins:** It's often possible to get all the clothes you need for free by asking friends and family, who are usually desperate to get rid of them. Go big on vests and babygros and think about the time of year your baby will be born. It's no good finding all the 3–6 month clothes you have are suitable for December if your baby will be that age in the summer.

4. **Nappies:** Not too many, in case you have a big/small baby and need to change size. Washables work out cheaper in the long term but are more of a time investment.

65

5. **Maternity essentials for you:** Maternity towels, breastpads, big, comfy pants.

6. If you are **breastfeeding** you'll need **a couple of nursing bras** (borrow if possible, and don't invest in expensive ones before birth as your breasts may change size), but don't buy a breast pump until you know you need one. Borrow a breastfeeding pillow if you want one – many women find them useful for a few days but not beyond.

7. **Nipple cream:** In the early weeks many women find applying a nipple cream to keep the area well moisturized can significantly help with discomfort and any potential damage, but breast milk itself does a great job too.

8. If you are **formula feeding** you will need 6 bottles (buy more later if you find you need them), teats, a sterilizer (10 minutes in a pan of boiling water works, but can be more of a faff than a cheap, second-hand steam sterilizer) and formula. The cheapest formula is essentially the same as the most expensive.

9. **A changing mat and wipes**: Washable wipes are brilliant and cheaper in the long-term if you can get over your initial scepticism.

If you need to add to this list, do. Feel good about buying what helps you feel ready and excited.

Be shopping savvy

- Remember that THE SHOPS WILL STILL BE OPEN AFTER BIRTH. Buy only what you need now – this isn't an apocalyptic panic-buying situation. If you find you need something you haven't got, you can usually have it delivered to your door within 24 hours.

- Ask for vouchers instead of baby gifts you don't need, so you can use family and friends' generosity when you need it later on and not end up with 5 useless cuddly rabbits.

- Don't forget to fill in your FW8 form, which gives you access to free prescriptions until your baby is 12 months. And now's the time to register with an NHS dentist if you haven't already. Dental treatment is free when you are pregnant and until a year after your baby is born.

- Organizations like Baby Basics provide free bundles of baby equipment to women who can't afford to purchase them.

- If you are on benefits you may be eligible for a £500 Sure Start Maternity Grant. This one-off payment can help towards the costs of getting set up for your baby's arrival, but is only for first-time parents unless this is a multiple pregnancy.

- If you are under 18 and/or receiving benefits you might be eligible for vouchers from the Healthy Start scheme. You'll get these weekly and can spend them only on milk, fruit and vegetables and infant formula milk.

- Remember that you can claim child benefit (currently around £20 a week for your eldest child) from when your baby is born.

Travel and adventure

" Patsy (my mum): 'I took great pleasure in striding past slow groups of men walking up Snowdon when I was 7½ months pregnant with you.' **"**

Women can have, do have and have always had busy, thrilling and exciting lives when pregnant. I didn't walk up Snowdon but I did take similar pleasure in marching up escalators, massive bump leading the way. If you are feeling up for it there's no reason you can't do a Serena Williams and win an Australian grand slam in the first 2 months of your pregnancy. Or whatever your own version of a grand slam is.

If your pregnancy is going well and you feel like doing it, you can fly on planes (hell, you can fly planes), go to hot or cold places, climb mountains, win races and see the world. You'll want to weigh up any risks and consider how you'll get any antenatal care you want if you are away, but you'll still get to have fun.

Check with your airline on their rules about pregnancy before you fly, and do consider how pregnant you'll be when you return. Usually you can fly with no bother up to 28 weeks. From 28 weeks most airlines will require a 'fit to fly' letter from your doctor or midwife, and from around 36 weeks (earlier with a multiple pregnancy) they won't want you on board.

Chapter 5

Your Rights

The right to touch one's toes or have a full night's sleep may be on a pregnant pause right now, but when it comes to your fundamental human rights, your pregnancy makes no difference.

If you are feeling pressure to do things a certain way, aren't getting support for your pregnancy or birth choices or have had a previously traumatic birth, it can be really reassuring and empowering to know exactly what your rights are and how to ensure that they are respected. Midwives and doctors are there to support and care for you. They joined a caring profession to help protect and uplift you, though sometimes the pressures of a busy system can make it tricky. So while you shouldn't expect a battle to ensure your rights are respected, and will likely find huge compassion and support, it is pretty empowering to know that the law is on your side, that nobody can make you do anything you don't want to, and that you always have the last word in any decision.

You don't need to be a lawyer, have a degree, and be good at writing letters or giving speeches to understand and make use of this stuff. At its heart it's about ensuring you are treated as the same reasonably rational human person you were before you were pregnant. These are just some tools to help.

So what are your most important rights in pregnancy and childbirth?

- Every woman has a right to receive safe and appropriate maternity care.
- Every woman has a right to maternity care that respects her fundamental human dignity.
- Every woman has a right to privacy and confidentiality.
- Every woman is free to make choices about her own pregnancy and childbirth, even if her caregivers do not agree with her.
- Every woman has a right to equality and freedom from discrimination.

Where do these rights come from?

Happily for all of you, you don't have to take my word for it. Your rights are protected by international and national laws, conventions and treaties – from the Universal Declaration of Human Rights to our own legal cases – and are further set out in long-standing government policy and the professional codes of the midwives and doctors who care for you. But what does that look like in practice and what does it mean for you?

Do I have a right to choose where I give birth?

In a word, yes! The law protects your right to decide where to give birth and you cannot be forced to give birth somewhere you don't want to.

All women in the UK are legally entitled to give birth in hospital (see page 183 for more on hospital birth). For the vast majority of us, this care is given for free. Some women who aren't ordinarily residents of the UK may be charged for their maternity care, but regardless of your ability to pay, if you need treatment you should be looked after first and charged later.

All areas are also expected by the government to have out-of-hospital facilities available for you, including birth centres (see page 186 for more about birth centres) and home birth services (see page 190 for more about home birth). If you don't have these facilities in your local area, you can refer yourself to another area or ask your GP to refer you. If you have any problems booking in with a trust or hospital of your choosing, you'll find guidance and support on the Birthrights website, www.birthrights.org.uk.

Birth centres often have guidelines on who they will accept and who is considered too complex a case. It's important to remember that these are guidelines, not rules, that they often differ from one area to another and that they aren't always tied to the best available evidence. Some women (for example those with a higher BMI, or who have had more than 5 babies, or are over 40) are outside the guidelines for some birth centres. However, many women feel that their chance of having the birth that they feel is best for them or their baby will be maximized by being in a birth centre. It's reassuring to know that many birth centres can and do open their doors to women who officially fall outside their guidelines but who, after an in-depth chat about the risks and benefits, believe it's the best place for them.

If you don't fit the 'criteria' (for example if you are a couple of BMI points over the cut-off point, or are having a VBAC, see page 208, but still think a birth centre might be the best place to enable you to have the kind of birth you want), then the team has a legal obligation to consider your request on an individual basis and only refuse it if they have an evidence-based reason to do so. See page 76 for tips on how to get your decisions respected, even if they aren't standard.

If you are planning a home birth, no matter what your circumstances, you cannot be forced to give birth in hospital. All areas are expected to provide midwives to support home births for women. The head of midwifery at your maternity unit should be able to help you if you are having difficulty getting support for a home birth. As with birth centres, the team will have official guidelines on who is most suitable for a home birth. If you fall outside of those they should explain the risks and benefits to you and offer you alternatives. If you still feel a home birth is safest and best for you, then you should be supported to have one. See page 76 for tips on how.

The dreaded patient mentality

It's easy to fall into the trap of feeling passive and inexpert in a medical setting or when talking to medical professionals. They have huge knowledge and expertise to share with you, but they also need your expertise on you, your pregnancy and your baby. If you find yourself struck dumb in appointments, make a conscious effort to remind yourself that you are in charge before each one.

Who has the final say about any intervention, test or treatment?

The answer is always you. In any circumstances, as long as you have mental capacity, the decision-maker is always you. You can decline any standard test, vaginal examination or scan. In labour the decision on whether to have a caesarean, a forceps delivery, accept antibiotics or have an induction always rests with you, whether it is an emergency situation or not. The vast majority of us want to take the advice, the information and experience of our midwives and doctors into account when making these important decisions, and the vast majority of midwives and doctors want to empower women to be the ultimate decision-makers when it comes to their bodies and their babies.

Your midwife or doctor has a legal obligation to explain any suggested plan to you in detail, share the evidence, personalize this conversation to you and ensure that it is presented in a way you can understand. You should always have time to make decisions, even in an emergency situation, and shouldn't feel embarrassed about asking questions and getting clarification. (See page 221 for my guide on how to make decisions in labour.)

What is mental capacity?

Mental capacity is the legal term used to talk about whether you are able to make decisions for yourself. The overwhelming majority of pregnant women and women giving birth have mental capacity. Being in labour doesn't affect your legal capacity to make decisions (though as we discuss on page 170, it can make it a bit trickier). Most mental illnesses don't impact on your mental capacity unless they are very severe, and even women with profound learning disabilities have been judged by the courts to have the mental capacity to make decisions about their care in pregnancy and birth.

Do I have to agree to a caesarean if the doctor, midwife or my partner thinks it's best?

Nope. As with all decisions, this is entirely up to you.

Do I have to have a vaginal birth if the doctor, midwife or my partner thinks it's best or can I request a caesarean?

Birthrights often supports women having difficulty getting the caesarean they feel they need. If there is a medical need for a caesarean section then this must be performed as needed or it could be considered medical negligence. A recent legal case set an important precedent that, if there is an increased risk to the woman or foetus from a vaginal birth, she must be offered a caesarean.

If you are requesting a caesarean for non-medical reasons then the hospital must consider your request properly, in an individualized way, only refusing if they have balanced all the factors and can show that there are good reasons for refusing and the effect on you is not disproportionately damaging.

NICE guidelines (www.nice.org.uk/guidance/cg132/chap ter/1-Guidance#planned-cs) on this topic make it clear that you should be offered counselling by a specialist if you are requesting a caesarean for non-medical reasons, but that ultimately your request should be respected. Individual obstetricians can refuse to perform the operation but they should refer you to someone who will agree.

Do I have a right to pain relief?

Yes. All women are entitled to care which respects their basic dignity, privacy and autonomy. Article 3 of the European Convention prohibits inhuman and degrading treatment. You can feel reassured that those caring for you have a legal obligation to make sure you get the pain relief you need. More on pain relief and comfort measures in labour on page 145.

Who can accompany me in labour?

Mother, brother, doula, husband, girlfriend, best friend — who you have at your side in birth is up to you. You can choose who you would like to be with you at this important time. At a home birth this is limited only by what you feel comfortable with, and most women prefer less of an audience! In hospital or at a birth centre there are likely to be policies on birth partners. Many places have a two-person policy and also only allow one partner into an operating theatre with a woman. However, it is always unlawful for policies to be applied in a blanket way. So if you have a need for something different, your request should be considered in a balanced and open way, and if it can be accommodated without impacting negatively on the care of other women or on the staff, then it should be. A legitimate reason to turn you down might be if your partner has been violent to hospital staff or if you are requesting your entire football team support you in labour, blocking access to the room for key staff.

Can I give birth without a midwife or doctor present?

Most women are very keen to get the support of medical professionals before, during and after birth. A minority of women want to limit their antenatal care and/or give birth without a midwife or a doctor present. Freebirthing can feel like a positive choice for some women, and you have no legal requirement to have antenatal care or to seek help from a midwife or doctor during labour. Unless there are other concerns, a woman shouldn't be reported to social services for making a decision to decline care.

If you are considering this because you aren't getting support for the care you need, have had a previously traumatic birth, or are afraid of childbirth, please do read Chapter 12. Freebirthing isn't a positive choice if you feel forced into it because of circumstance and fear and there may be a different way to get the support you need.

What can I do if I think my rights are not being respected?

Rule 1: There is no such thing as you 'have to' or you 'are not allowed'. Whatever the complexity in your pregnancy, your options are still open and your choices are yours to make. If you are having a more complicated pregnancy, or you have a 'risk factor', you may want to adapt your plans, but you don't have to if it's not right for you.

Rule 2: Get clued up. The vast majority of women want to get really solid information, understand the quality of the evidence that is available, and ask the professionals around them for their support and opinion so as to make the best decision for them. Write your questions down in advance if you can. Ask your midwife to talk you through your particular situation. Insist on information that's specific to you, not just hospital policy. Ask to see the studies, NICE guidelines and any other official recommendations that this advice is based on. You can find signposting to these and more sources of information on www.rebeccaschiller.co.uk/noguilt.

Rule 3: See the right person. If you don't feel you have the information you need, or aren't feeling supported in your plans, you can ask to meet with someone more senior. If you are under consultant-led care you will be seeing doctors regularly and should know the name of your assigned consultant. You will often see one of their junior doctors at your appointments, but for more detailed information and expert support you may want to ask for an appointment with your consultant. Experienced doctors often feel more confident supporting non-standard requests and will have a great deal of experience to draw on.

If you do not wish to have consultant-led care, you can decline this and ask to be seen by midwives only.

If you are seeing a midwife who isn't supportive or isn't able to give you enough information, ask to see a more senior midwife at your maternity unit such as the head of midwifery, or a consultant midwife who may have expertise in your specific situation. Many hospitals have specific clinics for women who have had a previous caesarean, who are diabetic or who have a high BMI.

Rule 4: Be clear. Remember that it is OK to ask your doctor to explain your situation in language you can understand. Make sure any statistics are presented clearly. The best practice is to use the same way of presenting statistics, so your midwife should talk either in percentages ('you have a 2 per cent risk of something happening') or, as I've done throughout this book, in relative figures ('2 in every 100 women will experience this'). A picture representation can be really helpful as you try and understand what the risk means, so ask your team if they have any statistics presented pictorially.

Rule 5: It's not all or nothing. If your circumstances mean that your midwife or doctor is recommending a different plan from the one you prefer, follow the steps above to get a good sense of what you want to do. If you decide to change plans, talk through how you can make plan B as much like plan A as possible. Were you planning a water birth? Your team should be able to provide a birth pool on the labour ward, and many areas have wireless, waterproof monitors that you can use. Keen to move around and be mobile? Ask them to bring equipment into the room from the birth centre. Are you happy with some of their suggestions, but not all? Work with your midwife to tailor a plan that works for you. Some women are happy to be on the labour ward, but want intermittent monitoring and no routine cannula. All these things, and more, are possible.

Rule 6: It's still up to you. This is really the same as rule one, but it's worth saying twice. If you get to the end of these

5 steps and still want to stick with plan A, your team should support you. A senior midwife or doctor should help your team on board with your birth plan. If you are planning a birth that isn't absolutely standard in your area (giving birth at home when you are over 40, having twins in a birth centre, not having a cannula in place if you are having a VBAC), then it's worth getting your plan agreed in advance and documented in your notes so that anyone caring for you on the day sees that you have already had the key conversations about risks and benefits with someone senior. This helps them feel more relaxed and enables them to provide better care to you and stops you having to discuss it while in labour. If you are having any problems getting someone to support your birth choices, see Chapter 5 to learn more about your rights.

There is more detailed information about your rights, how to make a complaint and an email advice service through the human rights in childbirth charity, Birthrights, on www.birthrights.org.uk.

Chapter 6

Your Decisions

❝ **Charlotte: 'I felt a bit panicked at first by all these options and choices I had to make for this baby I hadn't met. Then my sister reminded me that I make billions of pounds worth of decisions a year in my job, my brain hadn't been removed and that I could probably work this shit out pretty swiftly. She was completely right.'** **❞**

Discovering you are pregnant, however long you've had to bend your head around the idea, can feel like falling down the rabbit-hole of decision-making. A different world opens up. One you've heard about, but from a safe distance. It's full of new things, strange terminology and changing priorities. Making good decisions – that reconcile with who you are, the kind of parent you are discovering you want to be, the reality of your life and your specific circumstances and health – is an important part of getting a grip on feeling good about pregnancy and what's ahead.

In this chapter I will discuss some of the key decisions that you will need to make over the coming months. I've focused here on the tests, screening processes and other more medical decisions, but rest assured that informed and powerful decision-making is at the heart of every other chapter. From the tests you'll be offered to what you choose to eat and drink, these decisions are yours and no one else's.

Making decisions in pregnancy can feel like a huge responsibility, particularly as it can impact on the wellbeing (or perceived wellbeing) of your future baby. It's normal and OK to feel this pressure – and when you start to make these important decisions, have in the back of your mind that no one is perfect.

Decision-making in pregnancy is preparation for becoming a parent, so you do get to do this your way. There is no right or wrong path ahead. And while you are beginning to set the tone of the kind of parent you want to be, you, like all of us, will change your mind, change your plans and change course more than once. Setting off in one direction and finding it doesn't work for you is part of being a parent.

There is lots we can learn and apply to the rest of our working, socializing and broader lives from the experiences we have as parents. Decision-making in pregnancy can teach us a lot. So take a minute to revel in the fact that you are skilling up in this pregnancy. With every positive decision, every regret, every time you change your mind and change your plans, ask for more information, stick with it, stand firm or wobble, you are learning.

Tests and screening

Your antenatal care will start in earnest when you are offered an initial 'booking appointment' somewhere between 8 and 11 weeks into your pregnancy. The appointment will usually take around an hour and will allow your midwife to take a detailed history, in order to get a better sense of who you are and to understand the background to your health and well-being. This is also a great opportunity for you to discuss any key concerns and priorities that you have, and to raise any questions or get any information you feel you need. This is your appointment, and will be one of the longest, least hurried that you have, so you might find it helpful to write down any questions in advance to ensure you make the most of the opportunity.

Questions for your midwife

Try keeping a notebook to hand during your pregnancy, to scribble down questions as they pop into your head. This way, if you find your head full of white noise and emptiness during your appointment, you can turn to your notebook for a reminder. Here are some suggestions to start you off:

1. Will I see the same midwife every time? If not, is there a way I can?
2. Where and when will my appointments happen?
3. Who do I call if I'm worried about something?
4. When do I need to decide where I'd like to give birth? Do you offer tours or discussion groups to help?
5. What free antenatal classes do you provide?
6. What tests and screening options will I be offered?
7. I'd like to tell someone about my experience of trauma, violence or a previously traumatic birth. Who can I talk to and how will they help?
8. I'd like to get my notes from my last birth and talk to someone about them. How can we arrange that?

During this appointment your midwife will offer you a number of diagnostic and screening tests and begin the process of booking you in for more of these at various intervals in your pregnancy – if you agree. However these are presented, they are very much an offer, not a mandatory prescription, and it should be standard practice for your midwife to explain why these might be useful to you, and outline any risks and benefits as well as detail what any specific procedure or test entails.

The basics

At your booking appointment, and again at future appointments, you'll be offered a range of basic check-ups.

- **Urine sample:** Tested (in front of you) using a dipstick for signs of infection, urinary tract infections, protein in your urine (which can be a sign of pre-eclampsia), blood.
- **Blood pressure:** Tested using a cuff on your arm to make sure it isn't abnormally high or low.
- **Weight and height:** Usually measured at your booking appointment and used to calculate your BMI. You may also be offered measuring at other appointments. If you feel anxious about being weighed by someone else, you can weigh yourself at home and give the midwife your details.

Blood tests

Offered at your booking appointment and again later in your pregnancy. The midwife will usually collect the blood then and there and will ask for more than one tube. If you are particularly concerned about this blood test, frightened of needles, or if this makes you anxious, you can request an appointment with a phlebotomist (a clinician who specializes in taking blood) and you can request the application of numbing cream to your skin half an hour before the test.

You will be offered testing for:

- HIV, syphilis and hepatitis B, determining your blood-group and rhesus status, your iron levels (to see whether you might be anaemic and to provide a baseline against which to test you again later in pregnancy), signs of diabetes.

You might be offered testing for:

- Sickle-cell anaemia and thalassaemia. These conditions are particularly prevalent in some ethnic groups, and you are likely to be offered the test only if you are in one of the groups at particular risk. You cannot be made to take the test because you are in this group, just as you shouldn't be denied the test because you aren't in one of those groups.

> Get into the habit of asking your midwife which of these tests she is offering you. You are welcome to decline any, or all of them, and if you wish to do so your midwife can talk you through the risks and benefits of doing so.

Iron levels

It's normal for your iron levels to fall in later pregnancy, but if they fall below a certain level, you will be offered iron supplements. If your iron levels stay low you'll be advised to have a managed third stage (see page 217) and might need a more detailed conversation with your midwife or doctor if you are planning to give birth at home or in the birth centre. Some women prefer to eat iron-rich foods and take supplements such as Floradix to try and avoid the constipation that traditional supplements can cause. Try not to drink coffee or tea or eat calcium-rich foods in the hour around taking your supplements or eating iron-rich foods, as they can stop you absorbing iron. I'm sorry to tell you that the antacids you may be taking for heartburn also interfere with iron absorption.

Anti-D

I'm rhesus negative, which means I don't have a particular protein on the surface of my red blood cells. If I were to have a foetus which was rhesus positive in my uterus, my body might start making antibodies against it. It wouldn't cause this baby any problems, but in a future pregnancy these antibodies might be waiting to attack their sibling, potentially causing serious complications.

An injection of anti-D around 28 and 34 weeks of pregnancy and after the birth can help prevent this. You are likely to be offered additional injections (as I was) if you have bleeds during your pregnancy. I found the injections a bit painful, but I am a well-known wimp!

Anti-D is a blood product but it has been through a

rigorous screening process and is believed to be completely safe. If you are rhesus negative you should still be offered anti-D even if you have a miscarriage, your baby is stillborn or you have a termination.

Toxoplasmosis

The *Toxoplasma gondii* parasite is found in cat poo and in raw meat. This is why pregnant women are advised to pass the cat litter changing on to someone else, or wear gloves, garden in gloves and only eat cured, smoked or raw meat that has been frozen first.

The risk of having this parasite is so low that women aren't routinely offered testing. Early in your pregnancy your midwife will ask you some questions to see if you are at particular risk of having picked up the *Toxoplasma gondii* parasite. If you are at risk you'll then be offered a test to see if your body is making antibodies to it. If antibodies are detected you'll be carefully monitored and offered further testing as, in some rare cases, it can cause miscarriage or damage to the foetus.

Ultrasound scans

“ Penny: 'It was abstract until that moment when the baby waved at us on the scan. They felt like a person that I wanted to get to know. I had a secret happy cry!' **”**

For many women the chance to see their baby in glorious black and white on an ultrasound scan is one of the most important and exciting landmarks of pregnancy.

Scanning in pregnancy uses ultrasound waves to create an

image on a screen of what is happening inside your uterus. It's not a photograph, but an impression of what's happening within that allows you and those caring for you to make some estimates about how you and your baby are doing. You'll get a clear picture of your foetus by the time you are 8 weeks pregnant, but by the third trimester it's more difficult to see what's going on as your baby is pretty big. If you have a high BMI or your baby is in certain positions it can be hard for the scan to be done accurately.

Ultrasound scanning is now widely used at regular intervals during pregnancy. Across the world there is huge variation in how many scans women are offered and why. In the UK you are likely to be offered 2 routine scans, and more if your particular circumstances suggest that this might be useful.

Ultrasound scanning is widely believed to be a safe intervention for you and your baby, particularly if it is limited to what's needed for your medical care. There is some evidence that repeated exposure to ultrasound waves might be linked to changes in the foetus, with unknown implications. In response to this it's recommended that you carefully consider the number of non-essential scans, such as private and 4D scans, you have. The fun of 'seeing your baby' or reassurance benefits might be outweighed by possible risks.

A small minority of women choose to decline some or all of their routine scans, which, like any intervention during pregnancy, are not mandatory.

Viability and early dating scans

If you are unsure of your dates, or have been bleeding in early pregnancy, you may be referred for an early scan or a dating scan. This will look at the size of the embryo or foetus, provide you with an estimated due date, and look for the foetal heartbeat. If you are very early in your pregnancy this may need to be done with a probe that is inserted into your vagina, rather than one that is moved across your belly. It shouldn't hurt, but you can decline a transvaginal scan if you aren't comfortable with it, though in early pregnancy it may be the only way to get a clear picture of what is happening. The sonographer will explain exactly what they can see and how far along they think your pregnancy is. If they can't yet see an embryo they will ask you to come back in a couple of weeks to re-scan you. It may still be too early to see the embryo or it could be a sign that your pregnancy isn't developing normally.

The 12-week scan

Many couples use the 12-week scan as a confirmation of their pregnancy, after which they will choose whether to tell the world their news.

The sonographer will ask you to roll up your top and roll down the waistband of your trousers (a long tunic top and leggings can be particularly comfortable and convenient).

Your partner, or a friend or relative, can come along with you, and plenty of women take their other children to the scan if they can't find childcare. The hospital should be understanding and welcoming to your children if they need to be there, though it's worth considering how you might feel if there's upsetting news during the scan.

The sonographer will apply a probe to the outside of your belly and will use jelly to help it move smoothly across your skin. It shouldn't hurt, but they might have to press with a little force to get a picture. They will be measuring the size of your foetus and will use this to estimate your due date. They will check that your baby has a heartbeat, look for any obvious problems and will also look at the position of your placenta.

Nuchal translucency scan

As part of the combined screening test (see below), you will be offered a nuchal translucency scan during your 12-week scan appointment. The scan will take a measurement of the back of your developing baby's neck. Measurements within a certain range are considered normal, but if your baby has a particularly thick nuchal fold it may be a sign of a congenital abnormality such as Down's syndrome (DS). The results of this measurement will be put together with the other elements of your combined test to give you a risk factor for a congenital abnormality. This risk factor will help you decide whether you wish to have any diagnostic testing to give you a definitive answer as to whether your baby has any congenital abnormalities. If needed, this diagnostic test will happen later in your pregnancy, and you can find out more about it on page 91.

The anomaly scan

The 20-week scan is a longer and more detailed scan. This halfway-through timing works well, because your baby has done a significant amount of developing and many issues will be obvious at this point. Much beyond 20 weeks it becomes more and more difficult to fit your baby on to the scan picture. If you do not wish to have the scan, please let your midwife or obstetrician know.

This scan will take around 30 minutes, and the sonographer will take a series of detailed measurements of your baby's brain, limbs and organs. They will look at the placenta and the amniotic fluid levels, as well as plotting your baby's growth according to your estimated due date, to see if it is growing well or is measuring small or large.

If the scan picks up any potential issues you will be referred for further scans or tests and a discussion with a specialist doctor. Many suspected abnormalities spotted at this stage turn out to be nothing and, however anxious-making it is, it's always worth remembering that an ultrasound scan is not a video or a photograph but an impression. One abnormal measurement does not a diagnosis make.

This scan is also the time when you can find out the baby's sex, as long as you want to and as long as your baby is helpfully in the right position.

The combined screening test

In the UK women are routinely offered screening for Down's, Edwards' and Patau's syndromes. These are very different genetic conditions, also called Trisomy 21, 18 and 13. DS is the most common and affects people in a number of different ways, leading to a spectrum of specific health complications and learning disabilities. Lots of people with Down's syndrome are able to leave home, have relationships, work, and lead largely independent lives, though some are more profoundly affected.

Edwards' and Patau's syndromes are rarer but more serious genetic conditions with a poor prognosis. Many babies with these conditions will not survive pregnancy and only between 1 in 10 and 1 in 12 will survive beyond the first year of life. The effects of these syndromes include a range of very serious medical problems.

If your baby is diagnosed with any of these 3 syndromes you will be offered the option to have a termination, alongside support with continuing your pregnancy if you prefer. You can find out more about each syndrome by looking on the NHS.uk website.

The combined screening test looks at your nuchal fold test result, your age and the results of a blood test. These are analysed together to give you a personalized number reflecting your chance of having a baby with one of these syndromes.

Ninety-five in every 100 women will have a low-chance result – that's a lower than 1 in 150 chance of your baby having one of the 3 syndromes. If you are in this group you will receive your results by post within 2 weeks. If your chance is higher you should receive a phone call within 3 days and an appointment to talk through your options for diagnostic testing.

Do remember that screening doesn't mean a diagnosis. A high chance result doesn't mean your baby definitely has a genetic condition, and a low chance result doesn't mean they definitely don't.

Diagnostic tests

If your screening result means you have a higher chance of DS, Edwards' or Patau's syndrome, you will be offered a diagnostic test. This is the only way to make a definitive diagnosis of a genetic syndrome, so though there are some risks attached to the tests, they are your only options if you need to know whether your baby has a genetic condition before it is born or if you want to consider termination. There are two tests available: chorionic villus sampling (CVS) or amniocentesis. At your appointment you'll want to ask in detail about the procedure, the risks, the tests' accuracy and which test is most suitable for you. Non-invasive prenatal testing (see page 95) is available in some areas and also privately. This is not a diagnostic test but does give much more accurate screening results which can be useful when deciding whether to have a diagnostic test.

CVS can be done earlier (11–14 weeks) and amniocentesis a little later (15–18 weeks). Both carry a risk of miscarriage (between 1 and 2 women in every 200 who have the tests will have a miscarriage) and can be uncomfortable or painful for you. The results should be available within 3 working days. If your baby is diagnosed with a syndrome you should be swiftly offered an appointment with a specialist to discuss your options for continuing with or terminating your pregnancy.

There are a number of organizations that can support you when making this decision. Antenatal Results and Choices and the Down's Syndrome Association (see www.rebecca schiller.co.uk/noguilt) are very good places to start.

Jayne decided not to have diagnostic testing. Having her third baby aged 40, she had missed the nuchal test window due to a paperwork error at the hospital and didn't feel her high chance result was accurate.

'I felt certain that my real chance was low, but the only way to be sure was to have a diagnostic test with its own risks. We wouldn't

have opted for a termination so were happy to
carry on without knowing for sure. Our son
didn't have any complications.' **"**

Edie's results for Edwards' and Patau's syndromes came
back as 1 in 50.

" 'We had the termination about 10 days later.
It was too late for the surgical option so I took a
tablet that started labour. It was pretty fast
and – though I could have any pain relief I
wanted – gas and air was all I needed and had
time for. Holding him afterwards was important.
The midwives were incredibly kind and took lots of
photos for us which I hope I'll be ready to look at
some day. Termination was the hardest thing I've
ever done but it was absolutely the right thing for us.
I regret that it had to happen, but our decision was
the best one we could possibly make. Two years on
and I'm pregnant again and this time my results
show a low chance of any genetic issues.' **"**

Charlotte and Matt's second baby, Chloë, was diagnosed
with Down's syndrome (DS). Having been their doula when
their first baby was born, I was also there for Chloë's birth.

" 'The combined result actually came back as
showing that we had a lower chance (one in 155) of
having a baby with DS – but by the time we got
that result we'd already found out that Chloë
had a particular kind of heart defect that gave her
a one in two chance of having DS.

93

If we were going to have a child with a disability, I wanted to do my research, prepare as much as I could for what was to come. I felt as though we couldn't make a proper decision as to whether or not to continue with the pregnancy without knowing for certain.

The CVS procedure itself was a little alarming but it was over fairly quickly. A few days later I had a phone call from a nurse at the hospital confirming that our baby did indeed have Down's syndrome. We were devastated and scared. The next day I was too shaken to face anyone and had a long chat on the phone with someone from the Down's Syndrome Association. I joined a forum for parents of people with DS and asked them to send me positive stories about their kids.

We decided that if no other major problems were revealed at our 20-week scan, we would carry on with the pregnancy. The scan went well, we found out that we were going to have a little girl, and we felt that we'd really made our peace with the decision to continue.

I'd had an emergency caesarean with my first child, and was keen to try giving birth naturally with Chloë. She arrived very obligingly the day after her due date, in two hours flat from first contractions to birth. Rebecca knew what I needed (changing position, taking off my sweaty dress, putting my hair up) even before I knew it myself. We had two

wonderful midwives, who were totally respectful
of our request (in our birth plan) to keep the
atmosphere positive and celebratory.

Two years on and being Chloë's mum is pretty
bloody wonderful. She's an absolute joy to spend
time with and steals hearts left right and centre.
She is a funny, feisty, curious, affectionate and
fiercely independent little girl. She is meeting
milestones at her own pace and teaching me to be
patient and enjoy taking the more scenic route.'

Non-invasive prenatal testing

Non-invasive prenatal testing (NIPT) is a reasonably new, more accurate and less invasive test for a number of conditions. Until recently it was only available in the private sector, but pilot programmes within the NHS are ensuring that it will be rolled out more widely over the coming years.

You may be offered the chance to join a pilot alongside your standard combined screening test or to have NIPT instead. Before accepting or declining you will want to know exactly how the scheme works, whether you will get your standard screening results as well as your NIPT results, and how accurate the NIPT tests are.

NIPT is a simple blood test. It is not a diagnostic test but studies have shown that it is 99 per cent accurate when detecting Down's syndrome. It is significantly less accurate for detecting Edwards' and Patau's syndromes.

If your local hospital is not offering NIPT, it is available, for a fee, in the private sector.

Checklist

1. Understand the range of tests and decisions you'll need to make by reading pages 83–91.
2. Make a list of questions to ask your midwife at your booking appointment (see page 82).
3. If you have a high chance of having a baby with a genetic syndrome, get support from Antenatal Results and Choices and the Down's Syndrome Association as you make diagnostic decisions (see pages 91–5).

Chapter 7

The Unexpected

Pregnancy can feel like a 9-month-long series of unexpected events. Unexpectedly wonderful, difficult or just plain weird. I've spent the last 8 years recalibrating my expectations, realizing I was barking up a forest of wrong trees and confronting things I had never even contemplated. I've loved aspects of motherhood that I'd never even heard of. And some of my toughest experiences have crept up behind me, claws barred, without me hearing the lightest footstep.

Pregnancy is different for each and every one of us. And the same woman can find that her experience in one pregnancy is wildly at odds with her next. However deeply you prepare, something is bound to surprise you.

This is your pregnancy and it would be boring if it was just like the guidebook.

What was the most unexpected thing
about your pregnancy?

" Clara: 'That I loved my baby from the moment I got that positive pregnancy test. I was alone in Thailand when I found out and immediately it was like, "Well, there's two of us now."'

Layla: 'The shock of food aversions,
huge appetite and cravings.'

Kay: 'That EVERYTHING is affected. Hair, blood
vessels, skin, feet, moles, bowels, the lot. Even my
eyesight changed.'

Joan: 'Hitting 13 weeks and all the tiredness and
sickness disappearing and just literally glowing with
good health and anticipation.'

Liz: 'That pregnancy can cause carpal tunnel, making
it really painful to type. But that it would disappear
completely within about 6 hours of giving birth.'

Fiona: 'That I'd find it so hard to believe there was a
baby in there, let alone bond with it. I kept feeling
certain it would just turn out to be a lot of trapped
wind. I felt totally different once she was born though.'

Michelle: 'That pregnancy didn't make me vulnerable
and how important it is to be in control. That
automatically my body would dislike things that weren't
ideal, like the smell of smoke and alcohol, and I would
suddenly crave things that I previously disliked. Oh and
how incredibly sexy and horny I felt all the time.'

Cassie: 'How quickly you learn to scowl
ferociously at people who look as if they're
leaning in for a tummy rub.'

Kay: 'How many nosebleeds I had.'

Rebecca: 'How much I would hate being pregnant.
The first time I was in denial as though if I admitted
it, it meant I somehow didn't love my baby.
Second time around I openly disliked it and was
counting down the days to not being pregnant
any more as I knew I wouldn't be throwing up and
on the verge of fainting constantly.'

Francesca: 'How you are absolutely and utterly ruled by
hormones, and what powerful things they are – keeping
you happy and positive when the pregnancy comes out
of the blue, putting you off smells and tastes, helping to
grow that baby, turning you to a feeble mess any time a
baby or anything baby related comes on TV.'

Cassie: 'How hellishly tricky putting shoes on,
cutting toenails or seeing your "bits" are for
the last few months.'

Kay: 'That I could smell every single component of
bread. And cat food. If it wasn't for my husband our
poor cat would have died of hunger. Puke!'

Sarah: 'Symphysis pubis dysfunction – SPD. Who knew
that your pelvis is in two parts? And that when they
decide to separate 5 months into the pregnancy it
means that walking is impossible as it feels like your
fanny's being cleft in twain. Still hurts now, 8 years on.'

Reena: 'That there is no feeling in the world that
compares to seeing a positive result on a test
and seeing your baby for the first time on a scan.

Talk about magical . . . conversely, getting gestational diabetes was an utter pile of hairy balls! Just shitty genes meant my third trimester was spent having tests/stressing about food/pricking my finger after every meal/ultimately having a highly medicalized birth.'

Nilufer: 'That nobody tells you how painful your boobs can be in the first trimester. I couldn't walk because it felt like I was being repeatedly stabbed in the chest. I cried a lot because of those bloody boobs!'

Lucy: 'That being pregnant actually felt absolutely fine. In fact, it rather suited me. I didn't have to hold my tummy in and I could eat what I liked.'

Amy: 'That a singleton pregnancy wasn't any easier than a twin one!'

Jacqui: 'That I had a butterfly mask of pregnancy – splashes of dark skin that appeared on my face. Mine was mild but a friend had a very noticeable one which took years to fade.'

Una: 'That excessive saliva would torment me throughout my first pregnancy with twins.'

J'Nel: 'That I felt so strong and powerful carrying and growing a baby inside of me. Even though I was extremely tired most days, I still felt like I was doing something amazing.'

Millie: 'The restless legs – they are the most annoying things in the world?'

Mary: 'That even though I'm a scientist I'd find myself bewildered by the statistics and the decisions and how some medical professionals treat you like pregnancy has made your brain fall out.'

Nilufer: 'My undercarriage smelled constantly of digestive biscuits. I have no idea why but I couldn't get rid of it.'

Sophy: 'That I would feel so deeply content from the get-go. All the various money worries and other very practical concerns I had had over the years about pregnancy seemed suddenly clearly irrelevant to the very deep sense of joy that descended upon me. Some kind of hormonal cocktail meant I often felt almost high, and there were plenty of days I shed a few tears of happiness on my walk to and from work, because I felt just so overwhelmingly, thoroughly brilliant.'

Jacqui: 'All the extra ear wax! In fact, extra EVERY body fluid!'

Hilary: 'Not being able to go to the loo for 8 months. Nobody tells you about the constipation. Or its long-term results [haemorrhoids].'

Ana: 'That I couldn't stop farting ALL THE TIME.'

Lynley: 'Oh, I sneezed all the way
through my pregnancy.'

Vicky: 'My hormones made me accuse a stranger
of writing down my number plate for no
reason other than I was insane. Think I terrified
the poor fella.'

Francine: 'How much I would totally and utterly love
my midwife and how incredible the NHS is. The
anaesthetist, the doctor, the paediatricians – all of
them were fantastic!'

Deborah: 'That it was totally doable,
joyful and utterly amazing.'

Antonia: 'How big my belly could grow.'

Kate: 'That having always been a brilliant
sleeper I'd become a raging insomniac just when
everyone was telling me to stock up on sleep
before I had the baby waking me up.'

Lisa: 'That I didn't feel fat and my
husband still fancied me.'

"

Niggles, complications and surprises

You might experience one or two (but not all) of the unexpected pregnancy issues below.

Bleeding

Bleeding from your vagina during pregnancy can be frightening. For some women it can indicate the beginning of a miscarriage (see page 331). For others, bleeding can be a sign of a problem in their pregnancy. I experienced bleeding, some quite significant, during both of my pregnancies, for reasons that were never identified. It freaked me out, but in the end it just seemed to be normal for me. If you are experiencing light bleeding or spotting you'll probably want to get advice from your midwife. If your bleeding is heavy or free-flowing, go straight to your nearest maternity unit. If you are rhesus negative you'll be offered an anti-D injection after a bleed.

Pelvic floor weakness

Pregnancy and birth can play havoc with your pelvic floor. Lots of us experience stress incontinence – leaking urine while exercising, coughing/sneezing or laughing – during our pregnancies and after the baby is born. It's especially common as you are getting towards the finish line and your heavy uterus is pressing down on your bladder; meanwhile your hormones have weakened your natural control mechanisms. Fun times!

There's debate about if, when and how to do pelvic floor exercises. Do your own research but, on balance, it seems a really good idea for most women to do them in pregnancy and after birth. Products and apps can make this easier, and training devices that you put inside your vagina can help you get maximum results. Bog standard clenching exercises have the benefit of being completely free and you can do them anywhere – after practising your nonchalant face in the mirror first.

Here's a suggested regime to get you started. Remember to do these after your baby is born too!

1. Close up your anus as if you're trying to prevent a bowel movement.
2. Simultaneously draw in your vagina as if you're gripping a tampon, as well as your urethra as if stopping the flow of urine.
3. Start by doing this quickly – tightening and releasing the muscles immediately.
4. Then try it more slowly, holding the clenches for as long as you can before you relax: try to count to 10.
5. Do 3 sets of 8 squeezes every day if possible. Set yourself a reminder on your phone, or time them with each meal.

Sickness

Morning sickness is most common in the first trimester, often starting around week 6 or 7 and hopefully disappearing as the second trimester kicks in. Contrary to its ridiculous title, it does not just happen in the morning. Some women feel more sick in the evenings, or at lunchtime, and some poor unfortunates feel sick all the time, every day. If you haven't been told that eating and drinking ginger helps some women control their sickness then it's worth knowing that a) it can help some women with mild symptoms a little bit, and b) people will tell you about this again and again until you get close to shoving ginger biscuits up their noses. Some women swear by travel sickness bands, others have used acupuncture to help, and I found nibbling little and often was the only way to keep my feelings of nausea in check.

Your sense of smell may well be really acute, meaning that you can't stand your colleague's packed lunch or love the smell of a particular oil. Lavender, ylang ylang, neroli and rose geranium oils are considered safe in pregnancy. If you like a scent, consider carrying it around with you to mask the things that make you feel queasy.

Between 1 in 100 and 1 in 150 women will have a severe form of sickness called hyperemesis gravidarum, which can need hospital treatment. There are drugs available to help you but research suggests that some doctors and midwives aren't very well versed in how these work. The charity Pregnancy Sickness Support is there to help if you aren't getting the treatment you need, or if you just need an experienced shoulder to lean on.

Your baby's size

Some of us are short, others tall, some heavy, others light. The same is true for our foetuses, which are born on a wide spectrum of weight and length. As being very small, very large, or not growing as expected can be an indicator of potential problems, you'll be offered regular assessments of how your baby is growing throughout your pregnancy. Your midwife will use a tape measure to check the fundal height and will often feel your baby by palpating (prodding) your abdomen. Measurements will be taken at scans to estimate how your baby is growing and, if there are concerns about growth, more regular scans will be offered and the growth plotted on a chart.

A suspected large or small baby can trigger suggestions of an early induction of labour or, depending on your circumstances, a caesarean section. These interventions can be an important way for some babies to be born safely, but do sometimes mean that healthy babies are born earlier than need be, or by caesarean, which can expose them to other risks. As it can be really difficult to estimate a foetus's size accurately using a scan, you'll want to get good information from your midwife or doctor on any other signs of potential problems and complications before making any big decisions related to your baby's size.

Twins (or more)

Multiple births are on the rise, thanks to more IVF and more women having babies at over 35. Three in every 200 pregnancies are multiples, with the overwhelming majority being twins. Triplets and larger groups of multiples are now very rare, even in IVF pregnancies. You are more likely to conceive a bonus baby if you are tall or overweight, over 35 (and particularly if you are over 45), have had twins before or have twins in your family, or are Nigerian or of Nigerian descent.

Around 1 in 4 assisted pregnancies results in a multiple pregnancy, though guidelines are much stricter on assisted conception these days to try and reduce the number of multiple pregnancies – particularly triplets and more – which carry greater risks for everyone.

" Amy: 'If you are having twins, be as informed as possible and as realistic as possible. Try and speak to the highest up person you can, as other staff may not have the knowledge of hospital protocol to discuss aspects of multiple births. Ask "why?" as much as possible. If you hear "no", then get all the facts, figures and research, fully understand the pros and cons yourself. Then, if you still feel strongly, don't be afraid to take it further. Obviously some types of twin pregnancies have significant risks and complications and will require specific courses of action to ensure the health of everyone. If/when things don't go completely to plan during the birth, try and keep as much as possible of what's important to you. I had an epidural but was still active for much of the birth, we were in the labour ward but had aromatherapy and music, and we took our music into the theatre so it was playing as our babies were born. Immediately after the birth, my main tip would be to ask for a private room if you don't get one automatically, as they do try to prioritize multiple births if they can.'

Gestational diabetes (GD)

Some women aren't able to produce as much insulin as they need to cope with the rising demand in pregnancy and therefore develop high blood sugars. This causes a kind of diabetes that usually disappears after the baby is born. It can sometimes be controlled through diet (see page 26 for tips), but many women will need medication to control their blood sugars.

If you have one of the risk factors for GD you'll be offered a 'glucose tolerance test', which involves fasting for a period of time, drinking a sugary drink and having a couple of blood tests. If it turns out that you do have GD, your midwife will refer you to a doctor to talk through your options for managing the condition. You are likely to be advised to have more regular monitoring of your baby's growth and might be recommended an early induction of labour. You'll want to find out the risks and benefits of this for you, based on how you are managing your GD, before making your decision on whether to be induced.

Pre-eclampsia and HELLP syndrome

Six in 100 pregnant women experience mild pre-eclampsia, with 1 or 2 of them having severe cases. Some of these will experience a variant of this called HELLP syndrome. The condition is a serious one, and if untreated can lead to women and their babies being seriously ill or even dying. This very rarely happens, as your midwife will be checking you for early signs of the illness at your antenatal appointments. Symptoms include: high blood pressure, headaches, protein in your urine, blurred vision, a pain just below your ribs and fluid retention causing swollen or puffy hands, ankles, feet or face.

If you have the symptoms above, even if you don't have all of them or aren't sure, seek medical help immediately. Mild cases may be monitored in hospital, with medication offered to you to help lower your blood pressure. The only cure for the condition is for your baby to be born, so in more severe cases, even if your baby is not yet full-term, an induction of labour or caesarean section is likely to be offered.

Placenta praevia

During a scan, lots of women discover that they have a low-lying placenta. This means it has attached close to or covering the cervix. The vast majority move up and out of the way as your uterus grows. Only 1 in 600 women's placentas will stay within a couple of centimetres or covering the cervical opening close to their due date. If you are one of them, there's no sugar-coating it, placenta praevia is a pain. Bed rest or a hospital admission might be recommended, and you'll be advised not to have sex or do anything to bring on labour or disturb your cervix. You'll be offered a caesarean section before labour, as the dilating cervix could cause the placenta to detach, putting you at risk of bleeding heavily and potentially interrupting your baby's oxygen supply.

Digestion

Your stomach and intestines move upwards pretty dramatically in pregnancy and get quite compressed in the third trimester. Pregnancy can also stop the valve that prevents stomach acid tracking up working properly. Many women find they are constipated at some point (up the fibre, and laxatives can be prescribed if needed), heartburn is pretty common (drink milk, take antacids, sleep propped up, avoid trigger foods), wind and trapped wind and haemorrhoids (prescription medication and/or acupuncture) are annoyingly par for the course.

PCP/SPD

Pelvic girdle pain (PCP) or symphysis pubis dysfunction (SPD) is pain that comes on as pregnancy progresses, somewhere around your pelvis (front or back), spine or abdomen. It could be a mild ache or really limit your movement. In extreme cases strong opiate painkillers are prescribed.

It's not known why some women suffer this and others don't, but if you've had pain or injury in this area before, you are at greatest risk. You should be referred for physiotherapy if you experience PCP.

Your midwife will be able to suggest positions for birth that won't stress your pelvis further. If you have an epidural you'll want to make sure that you don't damage your pelvis by over-extending it when you are less aware of pain. It might be worth showing your midwife and partner how far you can open, bend and lift your legs before you have the epidural.

Baby's movements

Feeling your baby moving inside you can be an incredible experience. Some women find the sensation exhilarating and say that it helps them build a relationship with their babies. Others find it a bit disconcerting and alien-like.

In the early days it might feel like little bubbles popping or gentle scrabbling, but in the third trimester the movements can feel very strong. Sometimes, and especially if your baby is kicking in the same place, they can even be painful. Your belly might move, jerk or ripple as your baby moves around. If your baby is lodged in an uncomfortable spot, try shifting your own position to get them to alter theirs.

As your due date approaches, your baby will still be moving around lots. And though the movements change gradually through your pregnancy – reflecting your baby's size, strength and space for acrobatics – there should **never** be an abrupt change in movements and it is **never** normal for your baby to become much stiller than usual. Feeling fewer movements can be a sign that something is wrong. If you are anxious about movements, your maternity unit will be only too happy for you to come in, be monitored and – most likely – be reassured. Most babies respond to monitoring by suddenly putting on a tap-dancing show to assure you and your midwife that they were doing just fine, but early monitoring can spot problems before they become devastating. **If in doubt, check it out!**

Checklist

1. Expect the unexpected by reading what surprised other women (see pages 97–102).
2. Do your pelvic floor exercises (see page 104).
3. Know what's normal in terms of your baby's movements (see page 110).

Part 2

Birth

Chapter 8

Timeline of labour and birth

From 7 weeks | Braxton Hicks practice contractions are getting your body ready for labour – you won't feel them until later on, though.

In the third trimester | The hormone relaxin prepares your cervix, vagina and pelvic ligaments to make room for your baby.

36 weeks onwards | If it's your first baby, its head will drop into your pelvis, creating pressure on your cervix to encourage it to soften and open. This usually happens later in subsequent pregnancies.

37 weeks onwards | Braxton Hicks contractions will increase. You might feel more pressure in your cervix and vagina and perhaps some cramping. You may be hyperaware or unaware of these sensations.

Pre-labour	If you are feeling lots of niggles, or are having bouts of contractions that start and stop (often disappearing when daylight appears) you could be in pre-labour. See page 122 for more information.
Mucus plug	As your cervix starts to change you may find a blob of pink-streaked mucus in your pants or when you wipe – this is sometimes called a 'show'. It's been plugging your cervix but is no longer needed as labour approaches. Expect labour to start soon – ish! It could be a few days yet . . .
Early labour	You are en route to the real thing, but it's early days. You can still talk through contractions, they are irregular and short. Employ distraction techniques and alternate rest and movement. If you are having a planned caesarean you'll want to alert your hospital and make your way over. Some women experience phases of shakiness and nausea as early labour starts and again as it becomes established.
Home	Wherever you plan to give birth, you'll probably be at home for quite a bit of your labour.

Waters breaking One in 10 women's waters break before labour. Nine in 10 will find that their waters break during labour or the pushing phase. Babies are occasionally born inside their amniotic sacs.

Contractions The rhythmic tightening of your uterus that dilates (opens) your cervix in the first stage of labour feels different for everyone. Some describe it as intense period pain, others feel it more in their back or bottom, upper thighs and vagina. Six per cent of women in a recent survey described their birth as orgasmic. I've worked with women who experience their contractions as intense but euphoric rushes. Anything goes!

Established labour The official definition of established labour is 3cm dilation onwards. Your contractions will usually be regular, longer, stronger and closer together than in early labour. You'll feel less like chatting.

Water A shower or bath can help you feel comfortable and relaxed in labour – both at home and in hospital. See page 150 for information on using a birth pool for labour and birth. Remember to drink water during labour, particularly if it's a long one, and to keep urinating.

Pain relief | From breathing and TENS machines to epidurals, you can find out about the full range of ways to cope with labour on page 145. Whether you plan to avoid medical pain relief, or are keen for an early epidural, remember it's nobody's business but yours. And changing your mind in labour is fine too.

Transition | You might feel nauseous, shaky and fearful just before pushing starts (see page 127).

Rest phase | Some women experience a pause in their contractions between transition and pushing.

Pushing | It may creep up on you slowly, building from the end of contractions, or a sudden and overwhelming urge to push could hit. If you've had an epidural you may be less aware of these feelings, though the lower your baby is, the more you are likely to feel it.

Crowning   The feeling of your baby's head emerging can be intense or pass you by entirely. See page 133 for more information.

Birth   Whether it's smooth sailing or a bumpy ride, this is the moment you will meet your baby. Only you will know how it feels.

Chapter 9

Your Body

" Melissa: 'He was beautiful. Fat, soft and purpley/
pink and his face was super squished. As I stood in
the bath, feet in the water, babe in arms, I knew he
must be at least 10lb – he was actually 11lb 1oz! In
the days following, my whole body felt like an
enormous bruise and I felt such an immense
gratitude and self love. For all its pain and how
unbelievably mentally and physically challenging
the birth had been, I knew it was exactly the
experience I had needed and had worked towards.
It gave me great personal insight and was a defining
moment of my life. It brought together all of
my birth experiences and seemed to reunite
something within me.' **"**

Understanding how your body works in labour and birth
can help you make a birth plan that's right for you and maximize your chances of having a birth that matches your needs.
It's comforting to know that as we've evolved, our bodies
have evolved with us to enable our babies to be born. Nature
isn't perfect, all bodies have perfectly imperfect glitches, so
sometimes all of us need help with natural physical processes. But your body does have lots of its own tools and

clever tricks to help your baby be born and enable you to cope with labour.

Basic anatomy

The anatomy of birth isn't any old anatomy, it's your anatomy. And, just as our noses and breasts are wildly different from each other's, our pelvises, uteruses and vaginas all have their own unique shapes and quirks.

The diagram on the next page gives you an idea of the key anatomical players in pregnancy and birth. Your body will be broadly the same, but no one looks and feels just like the text book.

Getting to know your cervix

If you've never tried to feel for your cervix, have a go now. You'll find it at the back and top of your vagina. It will feel a bit like the end of your nose. If you've had a baby before it will probably feel a bit soft and shorter, with a bigger dimple in the middle. If this is your first pregnancy then it will be harder to find, longer, firmer and is unlikely to have started to open.

As the diagram shows, your cervix will start to creep forwards, soften and may even start to open in the last weeks of pregnancy. Those heavy feelings of pressure, little stabbing sensations in your cervix, occasional cramps and Braxton Hicks will all be working to get your baby in the head-down, low-down position that's ideal for birth and beginning to do the prep work on your cervix.

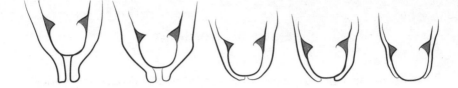

Effacement:
your cervix shortens,
softens and thins

Dilation:
your cervix opens from
approximately 0–10 cms

Pre- or latent labour and early labour

> **Louise:** 'I told Rebecca that I felt as if my body was fighting against these early contractions. Saying that out loud helped me to acknowledge the fear and tension I was feeling and I knew I needed to let go. At some point, Rebecca also said to me: "For some women, the first bit is the hardest." Although I don't think I really responded, this did sink in and I kept repeating it to myself in my head. And it turned out to be completely true for me. The rest of the birth was quick and much, much easier.'

Who knows when pre- (sometimes called latent) and early labour begin and end? I think that no one really does and that it doesn't really matter. In fact I'd encourage you to let go of knowing, caring, or paying any attention to any of the definitions of the various stages of labour. They can be a helpful, theoretical way to understand how labour can progress and what your body may do at different times. But thinking of labour as a pre-prescribed pattern isn't realistic.

Every labour, body and birth is different and your labour will follow its own course.

> ## What are contractions?
>
> Contractions are rhythmic tightenings of the muscles of your uterus. At first they soften and open your cervix by pulling upwards. Then, in the pushing phase of labour (see page 130), the contractions change to squeeze your baby out of your uterus. They are brought on, in part, by the release of a hormone called oxytocin. We'll talk about oxytocin again in the next chapter (page 161), as well as in relation to breastfeeding (page 300) and bonding with your baby (page 284). If you have an induction of labour (page 247), or you are offered a drip to increase the intensity of your labour if it has stalled or slowed, your team will be using a synthetic version of oxytocin.

Some women find that they start their labour by cramping or gently contracting on and off over a period of days or even weeks. This can be frustrating and tiring, so it's important to rest, eat, drink and distract yourself.

Charlie: 'I was so excited that I set the clock going from my first, tiny contraction. I decided that "this was it", lit the candles, got the music going, got my partner back from work.
Four days later and it hadn't really turned into anything and we were bored, fed up and tired.

Day 5 was when it actually happened – and pretty
swiftly after all those little runs of contractions
had done their thing – and if I'd just ignored
it as much as possible until then I would have
felt I'd had an 8-hour labour rather
than a 5-day one.'

,,

The upside of a long pre-labour phase is that your body has the chance to do quite a lot of the work of labour in advance: getting your baby in a brilliant position to be born, bringing its head down as low as possible into your pelvis to press on your cervix, and ripening your cervix. If you are having contractions on and off in the last weeks of your pregnancy, take comfort in the fact that your body is preparing well for labour and that you may find you've cheated some of the early stages. Second and third pregnancies are really prone to these niggles, even if you had a caesarean and didn't experience labour in your first pregnancy.

Any pre-labour should turn, at some point, into early labour. Alternatively your labour might start more abruptly without any pre-labour symptoms, with your first contraction leading to another, and another, in a swifter, more linear way until your baby is born. However your body decides to do its thing, those early contractions will be shortening your cervix and then beginning to open it a few centimetres.

Tips for early labour

1. Ignore it as much as possible, with the knowledge that this could be a stop–start process. You don't need to know what stage you are at or exactly when this will turn into the 'real thing'.
2. Think of ways to distract yourself in advance: walks, trips to the cinema (your contractions will be gentle and spaced out at first), box sets, getting a labour space ready as you'll probably be at home for a while.
3. As the hormone melatonin (which helps us go to sleep) works with oxytocin to facilitate labour, contractions often pick up when it's dark and quiet and die down when it's light and busy.
4. Rest lots, eat and drink. Labour is coming soon(ish) and you don't want to be exhausted. Nap in the day if you can – as your contractions may be stronger at night.
5. Don't be surprised if you spend a lot of time on the toilet clearing out your bowels. This, and some sickness, can be normal.
6. Feeling shaky and actually shaking can accompany various transition points in labour.

Active labour

Guidelines say that active labour starts when your cervix is 3cm open – but I reckon it is whatever it means to you. You are the one living inside your body, so you get to decide when you think your labour is really going places. A good baseline is that you will have been having approximately 3 or

4 strong-feeling, 1-minute-long contractions in every 10-minute period for an hour or so for labour to be considered active enough to need a midwife. There's a huge caveat here that labours progress at different rates, so listen to yourself and talk to your midwife if you aren't sure.

So how will you know if labour is active? You might not for a while, and that's just fine.

> **Caitlin:** 'I just suddenly felt certain that this was it after a few days of messing about. It was like, "Yup, this is really happening and it's unstoppable." '
>
> **Mary:** 'My partner said something had changed as I stopped talking and wasn't interested in the cakes we'd been making to distract ourselves. She said I had a glassy look in my eyes and didn't always hear her when she talked.'
>
> **Ayesha:** 'Very quickly in my second labour the contractions were longer and I felt like I needed to use all that time between them to get ready for the next. Over about an hour it became clear things were happening quickly. I wasn't pottering about the house like last time, I was actively working from very early on. It was time to go in!'

During active labour your contractions will continue to get longer, stronger, closer together and should become more and more regular. As the muscles of your uterus contract upwards they pull your cervix further open. Blood is diverted to the uterus and vagina. As active labour goes towards transition (see page 127) and the pushing phase (see page 130), that increased blood flow will make the muscles of your vagina work harder to soften and expand as your baby is born. Your body is getting your vagina and perineum super stretchy and expandable so that your baby can and will fit through.

Transition

Towards the end of the first phase of labour many women experience transition, an adrenaline-infused festival of intensity that tells you that you'll soon be pushing. It tends to happen somewhere between 7 and 10cm dilation and can last for a few minutes or a little longer. But, as the name suggests, it's a transient state that will end sooner rather than later. It can hit when your contractions have built to a strength and frequency that can feel overwhelming. The rest periods have become very short and the contractions are long and powerful, and it can feel as if you don't have enough time to recover in between them. It can be one of the most challenging points in labour, but is also a sign that you are nearly at the end. You'll spot transition if you experience some of these things:

- Long, strong contractions with very short breaks between them.
- Beginning to feel some pressure in your bottom towards the end of some contractions.
- Feeling or being sick.
- Shaking.
- Feeling afraid, overwhelmed and saying that you 'can't do this', 'want to go home' (if in hospital) or 'want to go to hospital' if at home. Many women also ask for an epidural during transition. See

page 147 for more on epidurals and whether it's too late to have one now.

Transition is different for everyone. Yours might pass you by – my transitions were very quick and not very noticeable – but I've worked with others who had longer and tougher ones that required lots of loving support to get through.

Tips for transition

1. **Coach:** Make sure your partner or birth partner has read page 178 on helpful things to say. If at no other point, you are likely to need someone to coach you through this bit.

2. **Reassure:** Remember and be reminded that this is a sign you are nearly there and will meet your baby soon.

3. **Normal:** The shaking and sickness is a normal response to raised levels of adrenaline that will give you the get-up-and-go to push your baby out.

4. **Now:** Focus on the now, one contraction at a time, rather than thinking about how long this will last.

Timing contractions and deciding when to 'go in'

I'm not a fan of slavishly timing contractions using your phone or a special app. It can distract you and your partner from working together on your coping strategies and can make you unnecessarily anxious about how things are progressing, as well as sometimes hindering your release of oxytocin (more on why in the next chapter).

> **Timing tip:** If you must time, choose a 10-minute window. Count how many contractions you have and time at least one of them for length. Do this no more than every hour or two to get a good sense of how your labour is progressing. But remember that you are the best guide. So if you feel that you need to seek support from your midwife and your contractions aren't quite matching the prescribed pattern, feel free to be assertive or ask your partner to be so.

If you are still happily chatting in between contractions, they are still quite short and you'd feel able to have a chat with some-one who came to the door, it probably is a bit early to go in or call your midwife. If your contractions feel they are coming one on top of the other without respite, and/or you're beginning to feel pressure (glamorously like you need a poo) during them, then you're cutting it a bit fine. It is definitely time to go in or get your midwife to you unless you are planning an unassisted birth.

Rest phase

When their cervix is fully open some lucky women experi-ence a pause in their labour. This is time for your body to rest and relax. If all is well with you and your baby, kick back, enjoy the break, nap, eat and drink something.

Not everyone experiences this pause, and you may find that the feeling of pressure at the end of your transition contractions just gradually builds until you can't help but push. Save your energy by letting that pressure build. You don't need to push until you can't help it. When it's time to push, most women will find that their bodies will tell them when and how.

Second stage or pushing

" **Kara: 'I'd learned this complicated breathing for the second stage. Cracks me up now, the pushing involved absolutely no conscious thought whatsoever. Gross analogy but it was like my uterus was puking out the baby whether I liked it or not.'** **"**

As you reach the pushing phase, the muscles of your uterus have finished pulling up to open your cervix and are now pushing your baby out. If the environment is right, and you are able to be left to your own devices, you are likely to experience the 'foetal ejection reflex', when pushing becomes an uncontrollable urge. If this happens to you, you won't need anybody to tell you to push – your body will efficiently and powerfully expel your baby. It can feel a bit like having diarrhoea – you can feel it, you know what's happening, but there's no crossing your legs or waiting until later, it's happening now!

Most women poo in the second stage of labour. As your baby's head descends it presses on your bowels and, though you may not be aware, some fecal matter may come out. Midwives are very skilful at wiping you and the bed discreetly and will be happy to see the poo, as it's a sign your baby is very nearly here.

Unless your baby is in distress, or you have an epidural on board, there shouldn't be any need for you to push until you feel the urge, and you shouldn't need anyone to examine you to tell you when you are ready to push. If your midwife is keen to get you actively pushing before you are ready, use the BRAIN acronym on page 223 to understand why and make a decision about what's right for you.

As you push, you might feel that your baby is coming down and then going back up. This can feel a bit frustrating, but it's very normal and is helping your body take time to stretch and expand slowly around your baby's head. This may be why studies have shown that if you are in control of timing your own pushing phase rather than following instructions, you will be pushing for longer but will be less likely to tear.

Pushing tip: feeling inside your own vagina for your baby's head can reassure you that what you are doing is working.

If you've had an epidural, you will probably feel the sensations to a much lesser degree, though the lower your baby gets the more you will feel. Your team will usually advise you to wait for an hour after you are fully dilated so that your baby's head comes down by itself without wasting your energy. Your team can then guide you on when, how long and how to push if you need them to.

Opening

I promised no bullshit, so this is the bit where I resist the
urge to tell you that your vagina is going to open up like a
lotus flower. I'm a bit less tie-dye than that, but the trouble
is – having seen quite a few vaginas opening up like sodding
lotus flowers – I'm stuck for a better analogy.

" Sophie: 'I just couldn't believe that my vagina was big
enough for a baby to come out and was pretty scared
about tearing. I tried hard to control my pushing
(with the help of the midwife) and she gave me a
mirror to watch what was happening. It was
completely mind blowing to see this little bit of the

baby gradually come forwards. All the fleshy layers
of my vulva and vagina seemed to peel back around
the head. My vagina was, after all my fears,
temporarily absolutely massive.'

Crowning

When your baby's head becomes visible to the outside
world – and it's often only a tiny elliptical sliver at first –
crowning is beginning. For some women it's the most intense
part of labour, but for many of us it's not. How you feel during this phase is really unpredictable.

Nia: 'I was expecting it to sting like hell, but the
whole thing was so intense that I didn't really
feel the head itself being born.'

Maisie: 'I felt increasingly like the skin of my
perineum was stretching and kind of burning.
It was a real grit teeth and wince through it
bit even though I had an epidural.'

Birth

For most women, their baby's head will emerge slowly. This
allows the perineum (the skin in between your anus and
vagina) to stretch gently around your baby like gradually
pulling your head out of a rollneck sweater. Once your baby's
head has emerged, its shoulders will rotate so that first one
and then the other is born. The rest of your baby's body will

usually shoot out pretty quickly and your midwife will help you to have your hands ready to catch your baby yourself or will catch it for you. If you are having a water birth, expect your baby to suddenly drop down to the bottom of the pool. It isn't breathing yet and is getting oxygenated blood through the umbilical cord, so you have plenty of time to reach down, find it and pick it up.

Keeping mobile

> **Hannah: 'Lie down on the bed? Couldn't have done that if you'd paid me. I was pacing, then on all fours like a beast. It felt better to move with the contractions.'**

Being active in labour, in a way that feels right to you and matches your physical abilities and the pain relief options you've chosen (see page 144 for being active with an epidural), can be really beneficial. Taking an upright position in the first and second stages of labour makes labour shorter, less painful and requires less intervention. This is often referred to as having an 'active birth'. Women also said their births were more positive experiences when they were able to choose positions they felt most comfortable in, which is a bit of a no-brainer. These benefits were still there for women who had epidurals, so despite moving sometimes needing a bit more thought, it's still possible.

As you're unlikely to give birth on the moon, and the whole point of this thing is to move your baby down and out of you, gravity is your friend; adopting positions that help your baby move further down into your pelvis by maximizing gravity's help gives you less work to do. In the first stage of labour, the further your baby's head descends into the pelvis, the more it will press on your cervix, and its weight (gravity again) will help encourage dilation. During the second stage your baby has to make its way down a twisting path through your pelvic outlet and into your vagina. Because of the way that your pelvis is designed, some positions can make the open space in the middle of your pelvis bigger. Essentially there's a bigger hole for your baby to make its way through.

How change of position changes your pelvis

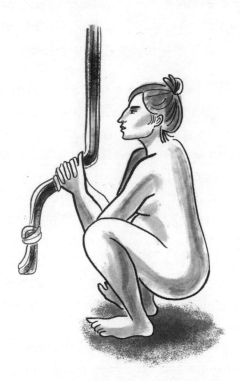

When you squat your sacrum is free to move backwards, making the widest space for your baby to emerge.

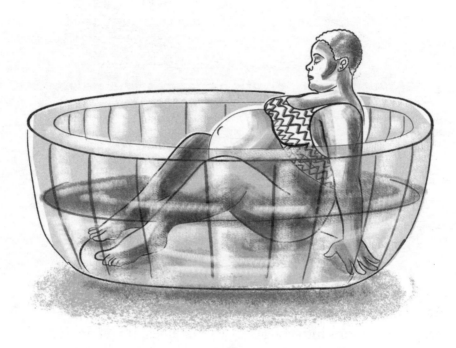

In a semi-sitting position your weight rests on your coccyx, making a slightly smaller space.

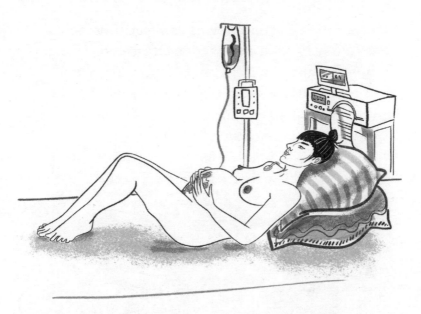

It is good to rest, but remember that when you are lying down your sacrum can't move and your pelvic outlet is at its narrowest.

Positions for first and second stages of labour

As your labour gets stronger, you may want to work gravity-helping positions into your coping strategies. If you don't find you are naturally drawn to a specific position (and I bet you are), try experimenting with a few until you find one that feels good. Consider the options below as a birthing smörgåsbord to choose from. If you have mobility restrictions, talk to your midwife or physiotherapist about adapting these for you.

1. Leaning: Try circling your hips, moving them backwards and forwards or lifting your heels up and down.

137

2. Pacing through contractions can feel good and help intensify your contractions. Place your feet hip-width apart, and lift your feet up, alternately bringing your knees up high during the contractions. Go as crazy as you like – this is a warrior-woman dance.

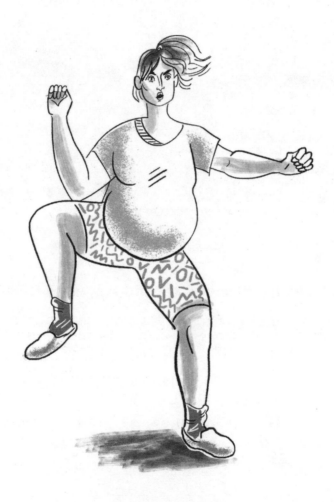

3. Sitting on a birth ball can get your knees and pelvis into perfect alignment and can take some of the weight and pressure off your joints. Consider circling, bouncing and rocking backwards and forwards on your ball. If you are tired, place it in front of your sofa or bed and build up a pile of cushions for you to rest your head on as you sit on the ball.

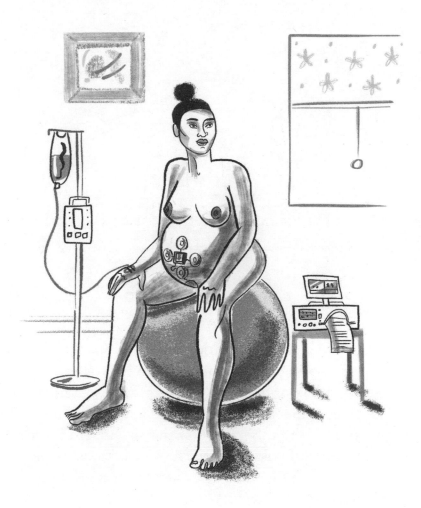

4. If you are out for a walk on a nice quiet road, consider walking with one foot on the kerb and one foot on the road. Swap sides on the way back. Make sure the road is clear – this unevenness in your pelvis can help to bring your baby down, but it's not worth getting run over for! Standing and placing one leg up on a chair, positioned in front of you and slightly to the left or right, does a similar thing.

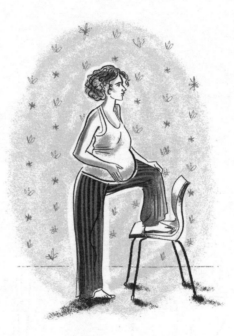

5. Stairs are your friend during labour. If you are trying to bring labour on during an induction, or intensify labour, walking up and down the stairs (during contractions if you can manage it and in between if you can't) can be really useful. Do it with a partner and hold on to the handrail. Try walking up and down the stairs sideways – two at a time if they are not too steep.

6. When you squat, your pelvis is very open. It usually feels very intense and is also tiring in labour, so it's something to use sparingly in the first stage but can really help in the pushing phase. If you need more support, ask your partner to stand behind you and get them to hook their arms under your armpits so that you can hang your weight off them as you squat and push.

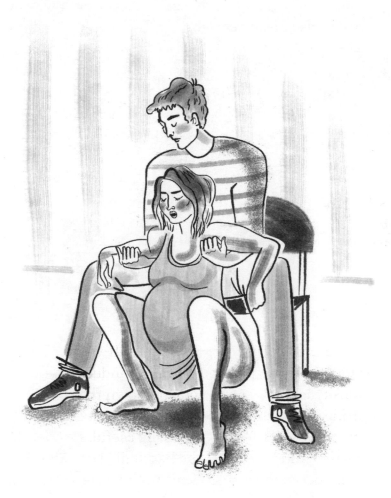

7. All fours, or more upright kneeling, is a favourite position for many women. You can be supported by pillows, beanbags or the head end of the bed so you can rest and, if your head and shoulders are slightly higher than your bottom, you are creating a really good environment for your anatomy to do its thing. If you give birth in this position you'll be able to reach down and catch your baby and bring it to your chest, with as much help from your midwife or your partner as you need.

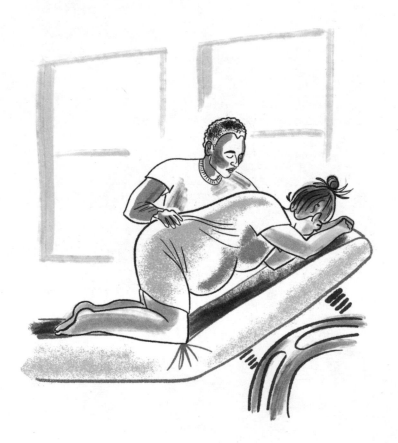

8. The 'whatever works for you' position: you may want to do none of these positions and come up with your own version.

Active epidural and resting positions

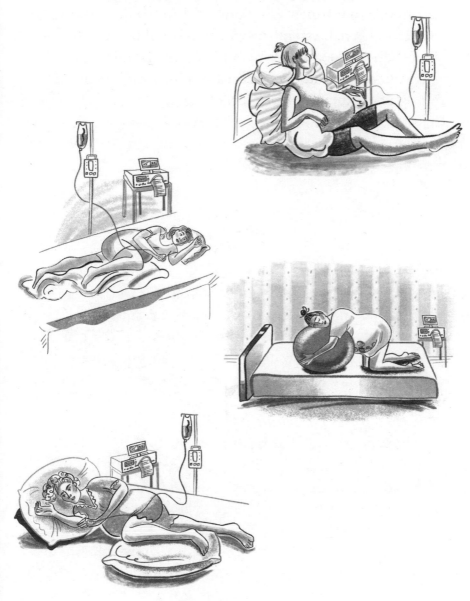

Active epidural

Depending on how strong your epidural is (see page 147), you can still be active with some help. Get your partner or midwife to help you try the positions on the previous page, using the bed, birth ball and pillows for support. A wireless monitor (see page 215) should be available if the wires get in the way.

If you feel very numb, ask your midwife and your partner to help you rotate through each of the four positions, spending a few contractions in each to ensure that your baby still has the opportunity to move around and get down in your pelvis.

Resting

Resting is as important as activity. You'll be exhausted very quickly if you try to spend your whole labour warrior-woman dancing, pacing up and down stairs or squatting like a maniac. Choose one of the four positions on the previous page, or alternate between them, to ensure you are comfortable while sneakily helping labour to progress.

Not being active

There are also some women who find instinctively they don't want to be active during labour, or who want to become less active towards the end of the first stage. I confess to being one of them. Despite feverishly attending active birth classes and my husband repeatedly encouraging me to move around during my labour, I refused to do anything other than lie on my back in the bath. He was a bit frustrated but I was adamant that I wasn't getting out. It turns out that I was having quite a fast labour and it wasn't until I reached the slightly slower pushing stage that I could be persuaded to move. Somehow I knew what I was doing even without knowing what I was doing. And I've worked with lots of women who, left to do what feels right and most comfortable to them, gravitate towards positions that are helping with the specific kind of labour and birth they are having. So while the positions above are a good guide, and I hope will bury themselves in your subconscious, remember to trust your instincts on the day. If it helps you – do it!

Pain relief and comfort measures

 Sushmita: 'My first birth experience was by no means pain-free but I managed without any pain relief. During the pushing phase I was in a trance, a sense of euphoria took over. It left me with a sensation I can only describe as "post orgasmic vaginal sensitivity" which lasted for a few weeks. I can safely say that I found it easier than anticipated.'

As you get to know more about the kind of birth you'd like to have, and also accept the possibility of things taking a slightly different route, it's well worth understanding what pain relief options can be offered to you in different locations and what non-medical comfort measures you can deploy to help you.

Let's start with the medical options.

Gas and air – also known as Entonox

Availability: In all birth settings in the UK: home birth, birth centres, labour wards, in the birth pool and even in the back of an ambulance.

How to use: You'll be given a mouthpiece and encouraged to deeply inhale the nitrous oxide gas during contractions.

Effects: You may feel lightheaded and distant from the feeling of a contraction. Some women get silly, talkative and even experience some light hallucination. Whether you like the sensation or not will depend on you. Many women find that it takes the edge off the contractions, helps them focus their breathing and means they don't have to resort to more invasive forms of pain relief. It can make you feel sick, but it is out of your system within 30 seconds of breathing it if it does. It can also make some women lose their focus and coping mechanisms and/or distract from pushing.

Does it affect the baby: No.

Opiates: pethidine, diamorphine or Meptid

Availability: Very occasionally at a home birth (but not in all areas and needs to be requested in advance), some birth centres and all labour wards. Some hospitals offer remifentanil, a strong, quick-acting painkiller given via a drip that you self-control using a machine.

How to use: Administered via an injection in your thigh during labour.

Effects: Are different for everyone and can last for up to 4 hours. It should relieve pain and make you feel relaxed. It can make you feel sick or out of control.

Does it affect the baby: It does cross the placenta, so it can make some babies slower to breathe once they're born and/ or have more difficulty feeding at first if they are born while the effects are still active.

Particularly useful if you are having a long early labour and need to rest, but isn't recommended too close to birth because of potential impact on the baby. You won't be able to go in a birth pool for a period of time, so check out the hospital's policy before having it.

Epidural

Availability: On the labour ward only.

How to use: Epidurals are given by an anaesthetist. Before one is put in place, or 'sited', you'll have a cannula put in your hand or lower arm so you can have IV fluids through a drip to stop your blood pressure dropping too low – a common side effect of an epidural. You'll be asked to sit down and lean forward (probably over a pillow) and your back will be exposed and cleaned.

You'll be given injections of local anaesthetic to numb where the epidural is to be inserted. The anaesthetist then uses a needle to insert a fine plastic tube (an epidural catheter) between your vertebrae and into the epidural space around your spinal cord. The needle is then completely removed, leaving the catheter in your back.

The epidural drugs are administered through the catheter. It can take up to 30 minutes to have the discussion, prepare and get the epidural sited (particularly if you are having lots of contractions), and up to 15 minutes for it to take effect. Depending on the system where you give birth, your epidural will be topped up by your midwife as needed or you can self-administer doses using a pump.

Effects: You will feel numb from the waist down to your toes. Modern epidurals are often called 'mobile epidurals'. These are a lower dose of drugs, allowing women to have maximum mobility and still be pain-free. Talk to your anaesthetist about how mobile you would like to be, but be aware that epidurals work differently from woman to woman, so you may be very mobile or your legs may feel quite numb. The more top-ups you have, the stronger the effect will be.

One in 10 women say it didn't provide a total block, and areas of pain still broke through.

You should be able to relax and sleep with the epidural and it doesn't have an impact on how clear your head feels.

Does it affect the baby: Mobile epidurals contain fentanyl, which does cross the placenta. There's some evidence that this could make some babies slightly sleepy at birth, but no evidence that this has any worrying effects.

Epidural myth-busting with consultant obstetric anaesthetist Dr Carolyn Johnson

Myth: There is a school of thought that, once you have one intervention like an epidural, you will then be more likely to have a number of other unwanted interventions like a forceps delivery or a caesarean section.

Dr Johnson's answer: 'There are large studies that show women with epidurals are no more likely to have a caesarean section than anyone else, and that epidurals do not result in any adverse effects on the baby . . . It seems from some studies that women with epidurals have a slightly longer labour (42 minutes longer on average), and some studies say they have a higher forceps delivery rate, although some studies also say they don't!'

Myth: Epidurals cause back pain.

Dr Johnson's answer: 'There are large studies that show women with epidurals do not get more back pain than women who don't have epidurals according to randomized studies.' See www.rebeccaschiller.co.uk/noguilt.

Myth: You can only have an epidural at a certain point in labour.

Dr Johnson's answer: 'It might be a good idea to delay as long as you can before you ask for one, as epidurals that are in for longer often cause women to lose more strength in their legs over time. You may maintain more control if you don't have it in for a very long time. There are no other medical reasons to avoid having one early.

There may also be some concern from your midwife or anaesthetist if you ask for one near the end of your labour, as it can be harder to monitor your baby while the epidural is being put in. More importantly for you, the same potential risks of an epidural exist whether it has been in for 5 minutes or 5 hours, while all the benefits in having an epidural are in having it in for enough time to give decent pain relief. If that time of pain relief is short, then the risk/benefit ratio isn't so good. This is a judgement call for you in labour, whether the benefit of pain relief will be worth the risks.'

Birth pools

> **Juliet: 'That [birthing pool] water is like some magic voodoo water. I can't explain why it feels so good and helps so much if it's just ordinary water – but it does. I've used it for 3 births and can't imagine doing it without.'**

Availability: Home, birth centre and some labour wards. Inflatable pools can be brought into some labour ward rooms, too.

How to use: Fill tub, get in, enjoy! Don't add products, as your baby might be born in this water. Water is kept around 37.5 degrees, and if you are putting a pool up at home, follow the instructions on cleaning it and using a liner and clean hose. Ensure you do a test run if using a pool at a home birth. You can choose when to get in and out, but most midwives will suggest that you wait until you really need the pool to get the greatest benefit and minimize the risk of labour slowing. If labour does slow you can get out again.

Effects: Relieves pain, increases women's satisfaction, studies show it shortens both stages of labour (probably because of the relaxing effect of the water and how mobile it makes you), may minimize tearing (though there's mixed evidence), helps some women feel private and safe, increases mobility and supports you through a range of positions. If you have a high BMI you may be particularly helped by the use of a birth pool, as water enables you to get into different positions and is associated with a reduction in the need for an epidural, which can be more difficult to put into larger women.

Does it affect the baby: No!

Birth pool myth-busting with midwife Pascale Hunter

Myth: It's dangerous for the baby.

Pascale's answer: 'Water birth is very safe for mother and baby. The baby has been surrounded by water while *in utero*, so moving into the birth pool is not like dunking their heads under the water. The water is kept at body temperature so there is not a big change for the baby to deal with. The baby is not touched while being born (so as not to stimulate any gasping reflex) and is brought straight to the surface by its mother or the midwife.'

Myth: You can't use a pool if you have any complications or risk factors.

Pascale's answer: 'You can still be continuously monitored in water if there is telemetry (wireless monitoring) available. This is becoming more common in units around the country, and birth pools are often available on labour wards. Depending on the reason for an induction, you may well still be able to use a pool if you are having a VBAC (see page 208), during an induction and in many situations where you have some complications . . . All midwives are trained in water birth – some may be more confident than others. All dopplers in hospital or home should be waterproof.'

Myth: I don't like baths, so a water birth will not work for me.

Pascale's answer: 'Even if you don't like swimming or baths, it's so important to keep an open mind and try the pool. We often get women who are unsure, and then they get in the pool and they love it. Be open to trying anything, you never know how you will feel at the time.'

Myth: Birthing pools are unhygienic.

Pascale's answer: 'The pools are obviously deep cleaned between uses (or new disposable liners are used in inflatable pools). If the water becomes dirty during use it can be changed. The midwives will also remove any large pieces of debris (poo, discharge, mucus) that make their way into the water.'

TENS machine

Availability: You'll need to buy, borrow or hire your own for use wherever you give birth. Make sure you get a special one for labour rather than one for back pain. You won't be able to use it in the pool (this would cause electrocution) or if you have an epidural (as your back will be numb).

How to use: Someone else attaches 4 sticky pads to specific places on your back (follow the instructions with your machine). There are electrodes in the pads, and wires from each go into a small control unit that you can hold or clip on to your clothes. Tiny electrical pulses are then delivered into the electrodes. You can increase the power of these using your control unit as your labour progresses. During contractions you can press a 'boost' button to deliver a stronger pulse.

Effects: Pressing the button and being distracted by the sensations can be helpful in itself. This can be particularly effective when used from as early in labour as possible: the electrical pulses give your body a head start in releasing endorphins (more about those in Chapter 10, page 166), boosting your natural pain relief mechanisms. They tend to elicit a Marmite reaction – you'll love your TENS machine, or hate it. If you are a hater you can remove the unit at any time, usually mildly electrocuting your partner in the process.

Massage

Massage and touch are an important tool for many pregnant women to have in their toolkit. Remember that some women find they want to be left alone during labour, particularly as it gets stronger. Massage that was eye-rollingly good in early labour can become deeply annoying or uncomfortable later on. Prepare your partner for this so you're not worried about hurting their feelings if and when you suddenly reject their tired fingers.

Exercise: Practising massage

- Sit with the person who will be massaging you in labour and talk through the kind of massage that you like. What pressure feels comfortable? What parts of your body do you like being touched? Are there any parts of your body that are no-go areas?

- In a win–win situation for you, ask your partner to practise massaging you regularly in pregnancy. It might be nice to massage them back sometimes too. First of all, try simply sitting in front of them, getting used to the kind of touch that you like. Head, neck, shoulders, lower back, feet and hands are often the places that are easiest to access in labour and in which we carry the most tension.

- Practise some of your labour positions from pages 137–43. What massage can your partner do when you are on the birth ball, leaning on all fours, or leaning against the wall? If you were lying on the bed, having had an epidural, would a hand massage feel good?

- Many women report feeling pressure around their sacrum (found in the centre of your body at the fleshier place when your back meets the top of your bum). You'll often start to feel a little uncomfortable around here in late pregnancy, so work with your partner to practise finding the place – on either side of your spine – that feels good when a little pressure is applied. During labour you may want to request that your partner presses firmly – being careful that they do not press on your spine itself – when your contractions feel strong. Many women ask for really strong pressure on their back as labour continues, and this can be quite hard work for their partner.

Other comfort measures

" Faye: 'Counting. I counted through each and every contraction.'

Brigid: 'My hot water bottle in my first labour and a microwaved wheat bag in my second – godsend.'

Joan: 'All the "sex helps birth" stuff I'd read about actually worked. Kissing and nipple stimulation made my labour stronger but easier. I didn't manage to have an orgasm (something about the midwife popping in and out didn't say "yes, yes, yes" to me), but touching my clitoris definitely turned the ouch into more of an oooo.' "

You'll find tips on breathing, noise-making and positions to help you cope with contractions on pages 174–6 and

137–43. Depending on the kind of labour you are having, the sort of person you are and what you have available, almost anything can help you in labour. Try it and, if it works for you, do it!

Checklist

1. Read pages 121–2 to make sure that you and your partner understand the anatomy of birth and the phases your labour may go through.
2. Make a plan for early labour, with things to distract yourself (see page 125).
3. Get your partner to read page 127 so they can support you through transition.
4. Practise the positions on pages 137–43 with your partner. Practise massage (page 153) and see which positions and massage feel good to you. Do this more than once, so you can both remember on the big day.
5. Think about what pain relief and comfort measures are right for you and talk through any options you aren't sure about with your midwife. Make sure that anything you need for comfort (hot water bottle, TENS machine, birth pool) is tested in advance and that you and your partner know how to use them.

Chapter 10

Your Mind

"

Helen's story:

'Somewhere deep down I knew there was such a thing
as a quiet, calm birth. But my first traumatic birth
experience had made me a bit of a diehard cynic.

My favourite affirmation, inspired by the Hippocratic
oath, summed up my plan for when contractions began
in my second birth: "first do nothing". I repeated it again
and again. I knew I'd need to feel as though we'd done
all the prep we could and then it would be OK for me to
switch my mind off and let my body do the talking.

The birth room had been readied with what
felt like every device and alternative therapy
save creating a life-size replica of a baobab
birthing tree in papier mâché.

At 3 a.m. I woke up feeling the need to practise
my breathing – this was it. By 6 a.m. I realized it
was time to get serious and deploy the birth
ball and ohmmmming. Cue enough candles to
power Birmingham for a week of power cuts.

This, my friends, was kick-off and I was
going in with open arms.

The contractions were now coming thick and fast,
but instead of the panic that I'd felt first time around,
I felt really pleased that things were progressing. I'd
requested no vaginal exams, not believing for a
moment that I'd be confident enough on the day to
go through with it, but I was and I totally knew what
was happening without them.

By about 7.30 a.m., I could tell that I needed to be in
the birth pool – and quickly. Bliss! 30 minutes later, I
was feeling pressure. I had my first and only moment
of doubt as I was transitioning. It didn't last and I was
soon into the only bit of it all that I would describe as
toe-curling. Incredibly powerful contractions were
washing over me and I could feel that the baby was
well on its way down. Even though all these
sensations were new to me, as I'd been numb for this
bit first time around, I knew it was all OK.

My birthing body went into hyperdrive now and my
primitive mind completely and utterly took over. My
body was pushing and there wasn't a thing I could do
about it. With the midwives hurriedly putting on
their gloves, my husband close by and me doing
some impromptu and somewhat random Mr Miyagi
arm motions to control my breathing (hey, whatever
works, right?!), I knelt upright and with one last
relatively easy push (only about the fifth in total,
I think) Beatrice was born. 7lb 12oz.

This is my proudest ever achievement, despite rocketing to the pinnacle of a flaming career in IT management (ahem) before giving up work to be a full-time mum. I am Helen of Troy, emerging battle-scarred, weary yet triumphant from my second birth.'**"**

Breathing practice 2: Equal and unequal breathing

This practice encourages a sense of steadiness and calm, and is the basis for the labour breathing practice on page 174.

1. Close your eyes (if that feels OK for you). Breathe normally, in through your nose and out through your mouth.
2. After a couple of breath cycles (in, then out), count in your head to see how many seconds your inhalation takes. Then try to get your exhalation to match it in length.
3. Do this for 3–5 breath cycles, counting each time.
4. In your next breath cycle, try to lengthen your exhalation so that it is one count longer than the inhalation.
5. Then try to make your exhalation 2 counts longer than the inhalation. And then in the next cycle, make it 3 counts longer.
6. Continue for at least 3–5 cycles, or as long as feels comfortable.
7. Before you open your eyes and finish, do 3 normal breaths.

Giving birth is an experience that has gained an almost mythical status. For many of us this mysterious leap into the unknown is something that we can't help but attach expectation and significance to. Historically it has been one of the biggest rites of passage for women, and we still carry the weight of some of that pressure today. Now there are other pressures too: hopes and expectations – many of them shared large in magazines, social media and on TV. For a range of complicated reasons many of us still, consciously or unconsciously, consider how, when and where we give birth to be a really important part of our journey to becoming a mother.

For those of you who haven't given birth before, the thought of what's ahead can be both frightening and exciting. And when getting used to the idea of giving birth for the first time, it's easy to only focus on the physical. What will it feel like? Will it be painful? How painful? How will the baby eventually end up exiting my body? Will my body work? And will it be forever changed by childbirth?

Birth in films, TV and the media doesn't do much to calm and reassure. Waters break in a tsunami-like gush, there's heavy breathing, screaming and machines attached to the woman's body. Often our only glimpses of birth before we have to do it ourselves are edited for maximum drama or controversy. It can be hard to get an honest, non-sales-pitchy, everyday view of what your birth might be like.

Giving birth is about much more than your body, and for most women it doesn't have to be high drama. Your mind plays a pivotal role in governing the physical process. You can use this knowledge to tailor your birth plan to work well for you, prepare your mind for the best birth possible, and cope in labour if plans need to change.

Everything I think

Spend 10 minutes, with your partner if you have one, writing down everything you can think of about childbirth and becoming a parent. Include what you know, your hopes, fears, stories from friends – anything that comes to mind. This can be bullet points, random words or sentences. Don't think carefully about it and don't stop writing – just let the words pour out. If you run out of ideas, write 'blah blah blah' until something else comes to mind. Nothing is off limits, too weird or too funny. When you think you have finished, make yourself write one more thing. Then swap papers with your partner and read each other's aloud. Tell your partner what you think about their writing. Do the contents surprise you? Is there any common ground between the two? Are you surprised by what you wrote? And does it give you any ideas for what kind of birth you want and what your hopes and fears may be?

Oxytocin and labour

> Emily: 'I retreated. Bits of me shut off like I was pulling out fuses. What was left was basic, primitive, and it was all I needed. Whenever I got disturbed and one of those fuses got plugged back in I was suddenly aware of it being painful. In my basic state I just went with it.'

It would be super helpful if I could start this section by telling you exactly what triggers the start of labour. But sadly, whatever magic kickstarts childbirth is still eluding medical science. Some have suggested it's the size of the baby's head in relation to your pelvis, other theories include a response to chemicals secreted by the baby's lungs in readiness for birth. It's probably a complex combination, but, as yet, no one really knows.

Whatever actually presses the 'go' button, science has given us a good understanding of the interplay between your hormones and anatomy that will drive your labour forward once it has begun. I'll give you an overview here, which I'd encourage you to read even if you are planning a caesarean section, as you may need to cope with early labour on your way into the hospital.

As we learned in the previous chapter, the labour and birth process softens, shortens and eventually opens the cervix, moves the baby through this newly opened passage, through the vagina and eventually into the outside world and your arms.

You'll already be familiar with the hormone oxytocin – the hormone that tells the muscles of your uterus to contract. What I've left out until now is that oxytocin also moonlights as the 'hormone of love'. Alongside its practical role in getting your muscles to squeeze, oxytocin is the hormone your brain releases when you are falling in love with a partner and when you have sex – particularly when you orgasm. If you love chocolate, you'll release oxytocin as you eat it, and the things you enjoy in your work, relationships and hobbies will cause your oxytocin levels to rise. As we'll discuss more in Chapter 17, it also plays its part in helping you fall in love with your baby and in breastfeeding.

Researchers are only just beginning to really explore the

role and scope of oxytocin in how we live, love, make friends, make relationships and connect with each other. But we do know it's secreted by the posterior part of the pituitary gland and seems to have different effects depending on the person and the context – potentially strengthening relationships with those you already feel attached to and distancing you from others. The classic and most documented responses to raised levels of oxytocin – and the most useful in the birth context – include feelings of connection, calm, openness and happiness.

The irrefutable link between our minds and our bodies is underlined by the role oxytocin has in labour, birth and new motherhood. And while there are some suggestions for further reading on www.rebeccaschiller.co.uk/noguilt if you want to geek out on birth physiology, below I'll set out some simplified but powerful information to help you as you plan the birth you want and need.

Exercise: Choosing your birth goal

Think about the very essence of what having a birth you are happy with means to you. Try to pare this down to one sentence. Choose a goal you can meet whenever and wherever you give birth. Try not to focus on where or how you give birth, but on the basics of what will ensure you feel safe and cared for.

Examples: 'Everyone is kind to me and I always understand what's going on.' 'I feel safe, supported and listened to.' 'We are all working together for the calmest, gentlest birth I can have.'

The oxytocin rules

You need oxytocin during labour to tell your uterine muscles to do their physical work to open your cervix and push out your baby. But oxytocin, being also so deeply connected to how we think, behave and feel, likes a specific set-up and is more easily released, in higher doses, if you are feeling a certain way. Want oxytocin to do its best work so that your body is having a regular oxytocin party? You have to understand these 3 key rules.

1. **Oxytocin's enemy is adrenaline**. Persistent, high levels of adrenaline sometimes cause oxytocin, and therefore labour, to stall or even flee. You may know adrenaline as the 'fight or flight' hormone. If you are anxious, frightened or panicking, your body releases adrenaline so you can fight your 'attacker' or leg it in the opposite direction. But our primitive brains haven't caught up with contemporary realities. These days we release adrenaline in response to a range of situations which might not actually involve the need to fight or flee. So, even if your 'attacker' is just you feeling worried about labour, anxiety about going to hospital or having an examination, your body may respond by releasing adrenaline. This could have a knock-on effect of inhibiting your oxytocin release and slowing your labour. Studies have shown that women who are particularly fearful of labour have longer labours.

2. **Oxytocin flows most freely when you feel good.** Feeling calm, safe, happy and loved allows you to release more oxytocin. Studies have shown that

women labouring in environments where they feel safe and comfortable have less need for intervention and report lower levels of pain. We'll work on what that means to you later on.

3. **Oxytocin is old-fashioned.** Ok, so it won't try to pay for dinner, but oxytocin is a bit retro. It's released by the older, primitive part of your brain – the hypothalamus. This is the part of our brain that we share with monkeys and other mammals. It governs our instinctive responses, releasing the hormones that cause our bodies to do things and our minds to feel things without any conscious thought from us.

   The good news here is that this means labour happens without us having to think about it. Ever wondered why animals seem to have an easier time giving birth? Some theorize that it's because they don't have such complex brains as humans do. The new part of our brain, our neocortex, is a big part of what makes us human. It allows us to rationalize, analyse, over-analyse, question, worry and debate. It is very helpful for making a decision about which route to take or arguing your case in court. It is less helpful in labour, when you need to be engaging the primitive part of your brain charged with releasing hormones.

Anything that switches on the neocortex (worry, talking, lights, feeling observed, making complex decisions) can impact on how well the primitive part of our brain releases the oxytocin it needs to. Think: monkey brain good, human brain bad.

An eye mask can help you block out the outside world as you make your way to hospital. Dim the lights in your labour room, or turn them off and use the side lamp, battery-powered candles (in hospital) or real ones (at home). Think about who is in the room with you and, if there are too many people, get your partner to ask anyone non-essential to leave. Remember, it is up to you whether students are there to observe. A shower or bath or trip to the loo can give you privacy and quiet if there's too much going on in your room, and a birth pool can help you feel private and safe. Ask your partner to do the talking and write a detailed birth plan when they can, so you don't have to engage the decision-making part of your brain unless it's important. Prioritize quiet. If your birth partner and you whisper, others will follow suit.

Endorphins

 Philippa: 'During my induction I could actually feel the endorphins coursing around my body. Up and down my legs. It felt incredible.'

In a labour that is flowing well, endorphins are released in response to oxytocin. Raised levels of endorphins (which you may already know from exercise or riding a rollercoaster) give the body a natural pain relief and a feeling of euphoria. In labour the body responds to the release of oxytocin by also releasing endorphins. These help you deal with the contractions and give some women a slightly spaced-out, high feeling that helps them go into a zone, cope with labour and shut out the outside world and its neocortex triggers.

Popular theories, which have formed the basis for many schools of hypnobirthing, suggest that feeling fearful not only has an impact on raising adrenaline and decreasing oxytocin (and potentially slowing labour) but also on the release of endorphins. The more fearful you are, the more pain you are likely to report, potentially making you feel more fearful, leading to a vicious cycle.

Exercise: Calm and stress triggers

1. Sit down with a large sheet of blank paper.
2. Start by thinking of your stress triggers. Write down the things that make you feel stressed in daily life. Think about work, commuting, relationship with your partner, friends and parents. Who are the people that irritate you, and why? However irrational that stress trigger is, however loath you are to admit it, write it down. Some ideas include: feeling out of control, people with whiney voices, when your partner asks you over and over again if you are OK, loud music, particular smells, feeling rushed, feeling under pressure, sudden changes of plan, people who remind you of someone specific that you dislike.
3. Now write down the things that you do, or that others do, that naturally make you feel calmer. Think about all areas of your life, and remember that none of these things have to relate specifically to labour. My calm triggers include: having a bath, rose and geranium oil smell, having a glass of wine, massage, specific music, being listened to, funny films and TV shows, my friends (but not all at once), things being well-planned.

4. If you have a partner, or a close birth partner, chat through what you've written down with them. Discuss any observations they have about what stresses and calms you. Sometimes those who know us well will have a different set of observations. If you agree, add those to your lists.

5. Now begin to think about labour and birth. Look through your stress and calm triggers and split them into 3 columns, marked 'location', 'props' and 'people'. Note down what you think you will need to do, how you can plan your birth, how your partner can help and what things you'll need around you to minimize the opportunity for stress triggers and maximize the opportunity for calm triggers. Consider location – where will you need to be (and it may be more than one place) in early labour? Will movement feel good? Is there a favourite pub or restaurant you could visit? Would a trip to the cinema to see a funny film help? Or do you prefer privacy? Might setting up a cosy nest at home be comforting? Will small spaces feel safe to you? Or a big one? In the props column consider the things you have at home and in your hospital bag to help you feel calm. These could include: photos, music, things that smell nice, a childhood toy, a particular pillow, an eye mask to block out light. In the 'people' column, work through who might be around you during your labour and whether they are the right ones. Does your partner appear more in the stress list or more in the calm list? Consider which friends and family might want to be there – are they able to minimize stress triggers and maximize calm triggers? Sometimes this exercise can give you a difficult decision to

make about birth partners, but it's better to know in advance that your partner, your mother or your best friend is more likely to wind you up than chill you out.

6. Talk to your partner. No one is perfect, and all relationships are built, at least in part, on compromise. Even the most sensitive and loving partner will have habits that drive you mad. Think about what you may need to ask them to be aware of and avoid while you are in labour. Can you sensitively make them aware of it and help them come up with something to say and do instead? Do they hum? Speak too loud? Ignore you? Play on their phone too much? Are they prone to ringing their mother at times of private stress or joy? If these things send you over the edge, talk about them now!

7. Use this exercise to come up with a set of your personal oxytocin party rules. Rules are the absolute things that cannot happen or must happen during your labour and birth. These rules need to work when you are at home, in hospital and however you end up giving birth. So steer away from anything as specific as 'I must give birth in a birth pool at 8 p.m. surrounded by singing unicorns.' Instead consider things that are absolutely crucial for you not to feel stressed. You might want to have a rule that you must always know what is happening and be in charge of decision-making. Or that your mother-in-law can't be there during labour. Or that you have access to a calm playlist even if you go to theatre for a caesarean.

When you have gone through this exercise, you and your partner should begin to have a better idea of what you need. When you've reflected on it more – and this may take you some weeks or months – you can begin to use this to think about where you would like to give birth. It can also help you think about any additional tools (hypnobirthing, doulas, TENS machines or epidurals) that you may need.

Shutting off your brain

There is a delicate balance between you being in charge of the big decisions during birth and shutting off your day-to-day brain to allow the neocortex to shut down. As you'll see in Chapters 11 and 13, I'm encouraging you to do your birth planning, decision-making, negotiating and as much of the new brain stuff as possible before labour. This will help, as it will encouraging your partner and/or birth partner to take an active role in protecting your oxytocin party when you are in labour.

You'll find it helpful to:

- Not to have to do too much talking. Small talk becomes old quickly, and when you don't feel like chatting any more, listen to your primitive brain – it's trying to take over.
- Not to have constant decision-making to do about what you want to eat, drink, watch and listen to. If you do end up needing to make big decisions in labour, see page 221 for my suggestions on how to do so quickly and efficiently.
- Avoid things which encourage you to have to start analysing and worrying, such as contraction timers.

Managing fear and anxiety

Most of us have our pre-labour wobbles. We can't aim to get rid of all fear, stress and worry. Life is full of all three, and becoming a parent is no exception. But if your fears about giving birth are distracting or overwhelming, if you have had a previously traumatic birth or experienced other related trauma, you might find it helpful to tackle these in advance.

There are many different approaches to releasing fear and I've included just one here. If you are seeking counselling and support for this, talk to your therapist or midwife about your fears and how you might want to tackle them. If you are experiencing symptoms of PTSD, seek professional help on how to recover.

Exercise: Fear release

1. Write down what your fears are. They might be profound: you may be concerned you will die or become seriously injured (this is of course statistically incredibly unlikely, but knowing statistics doesn't always have a calming effect); or they might be very specific: pooing during labour, tearing, or the pain.
2. Think practically about how you will deal with them. If you have a doula, talk them through with her. Chat to your partner and your midwife so that you have a practical plan. Then consider why you might feel frightened about this particular aspect of birth. Is it related to something that's happened to you in the past, or a friend's experience? Sometimes understanding where the fear is located can help.

3. When you have more of a handle on where your fear has come from and what practically you can do in your birth plan, before you give birth or after birth to help you cope, then you might feel ready to release some of that fear.

4. Write each fear on a Post-it note. Consider it, think through how you've dealt with it, and when you are ready to let it go (at least to some degree) choose an approach that's right for you. Burn it (safely), rip it up, throw it in the bin, or bury it in the garden. If your fears feel too big to get rid of, and your due date is fast approaching, you may want to put them into a box and put the box away somewhere safe so that you don't have to see it every day. You will know that you still have fears and anxieties but will also know that you have prepared for them. They are still there but are also safely locked away, controlled by you until you are ready to re-open them after your baby has been born.

Alice was having her first baby. She had dealt with some anxiety through her life and, after a couple of miscarriages and fertility treatment, she felt particularly anxious about her pregnancy and had specific fears connected to giving birth.

" 'I just couldn't stop thinking about things that could go wrong. My midwife was very nice and supportive. One of the things we did was fear release, though I have to say I was pretty sceptical.

We discussed visualization but that seemed too complex. Instead I wrote down my fears. There was something comforting about just having them on pieces of paper and not just buzzing around in my head. I wasn't ready to burn or bury them, so I just kept them on the living-room shelf for a while. Meanwhile we did lots of work to make sure that my birth plan was tailored around my fears. So I would give birth in hospital, had requested an early epidural and my midwife was going to try and be there for the birth. It helped to know these plans were in place but I still felt frightened.

About three weeks before my due date I decided that I couldn't erase my fears before the birth but I was ready to try and put them aside for a while. We put them in a cardboard box and I made a big deal of using loads and loads of parcel tape around it. I decided to post the box to my best friend who lives about 250 miles away. She didn't open it and put it in her cellar. I know it sounds completely mental, but I felt less afraid knowing she had taken care of these fears for me and they were – at least temporarily – not my issue.'

Calming and coping during labour

I want you to finish your labour feeling positive and robust enough to launch into motherhood. Feeling as calm, happy, loved and loving as possible (with the emphasis on 'as possible') is an important part of that. But instructions to 'relax' at a time that can be filled with stress can sometimes feel like another pressurizing and unachievable goal. Telling you to relax without telling you why and how could actually stress you out!

You will be able to cope, with the support of those around you. And some basic tools and techniques will help you calm your mind, cope with intense contractions and minimize fear and panic during labour.

Breathing and making funny noises

When I was pregnant for the first time I went to brilliant antenatal classes run by an experienced teacher and psychotherapist, Jessica James. Jessica didn't invent using breathing and noises to cope with labour – I imagine women have been doing that all by themselves for a while – but she helped us all learn how to practise a simple way of breathing and noise-making for labour. It has become my go-to coping mechanism for my own labours and one I practise with my doula clients.

If you haven't done the 'equal and unequal breathing' practice on page 159 yet, you'll find it useful to do this first. And remember – you're already really good at breathing and there is no great mystery to breathing during labour.

Labour breathing practice

Practise this before labour, with your partner, once a week from 27 weeks (more often if you can):

1. Close your eyes, if you feel able to. Start by breathing in through your nose and out through your mouth. Follow the equal and unequal breathing practice on page 159 to notice your natural breathing, make it equal and then elongate your out breath.

---

2. Continue until you can control a long, slow release as you exhale. There's no panic to breathe in again once your air has left your lungs, wait until your body does it for you.

3. Practise when you feel stressed, annoyed, are having Braxton Hicks contractions, or stub your toe. Notice the impact that concentrating your whole mind on your breathing has during times of pain, stress or irritation. You'll probably find that pain diminishes and stress lessens too.

4. When you feel ready, change your quiet exhalation to a noise. Experiment with a few different noises. They need to be low-pitched, not high-pitched (as this will make you feel calmer and encourage a relaxed rather than tense jaw). A traditional yogic 'ohhhhhmmmmmmm' works well, as does a low 'aaahhhhhh', 'urgghhhhh' or even a hum. Practise this with your partner, as you will both feel ridiculous doing it and need to get the laughing out of your system so you don't feel self-conscious about doing it in labour.

Using breathing in labour

1. In early labour, while your contractions are likely to be quite short and not too strong, practise the breathing when you feel the contraction coming on. Close your eyes and concentrate on taking in a relaxed full breath through your nose and lengthening your exhalation every time. You are just getting into good habits at this stage, so if you prefer to ignore the

contractions, breathe through a couple for practice, then breathe as normal until you can't ignore them.

2. As your contractions build in strength, focus even more fixedly on that breathing. It may help if your partner breathes with you, but ask them not to tell you repeatedly to breathe, as this is beyond irritating. If your labour goes up a gear and your breathing gets shallow and faster in response, train your partner to pay attention to your breathing and join in with you, breathing audibly in a slow and calm way until you are able to slow your breathing to match theirs.

3. When labour is really strong it may become more and more difficult to focus on this breathing. Now it's time to crack open the funny noises. You may feel self-conscious at first, but once it's helping, you won't care. It can help if your partner joins in with you. Make those noises as long as possible. Keep them low-pitched and your jaw soft. Go loud if you need to!

4. This breathing can be really useful when trying to keep still to have an epidural sited, lowering stress during a caesarean or to calm you before you make a big decision.

As your contractions build you might notice your hands, feet, neck or shoulders are getting tense. Doing the tension release exercise (see page 46) occasionally in between contractions can stop tension creeping in.

As your contractions get closer together you may not have time to do the full tension release exercise. Simply focus on areas of particular tension during the contraction gaps, taking a couple of breaths to relax those body parts and then, with a single exhalation, soften your entire body.

Hypnobirthing

Hypnobirthing can sound like mumbo-jumbo, but to me it is nothing more or less than a dedicated programme to help you learn how to stay calm, control your mind and give you specific tools to practise doing just that. You won't be walking around in a hypnotic state and no one else will be controlling you or making you think you are a chicken. If it interests you, you'll be able to attend group classes, individual classes, learn from books and CDs at home, or can do your own DIY version with enough reading up and help from your partner. Some hospitals provide free or low-cost classes as part of their antenatal offer.

There's still lots more for researchers to learn about hypnobirthing, but the evidence base suggests that at worst it does no harm and at best it may shorten labour, lessen the need for pain medication and make women feel happier and more in control.

It's important to find a school of hypnobirthing that's right for you. For some women this is one with a goal of a pain-free labour and an intervention-free birth. For others it's a tool in the hospital bag to help cope with anxiety, manage the stressful parts, and isn't associated with a specific outcome or pain goal. I confess to preferring the latter approach, as it's less likely to give you a goal you might not meet.

The birth environment

Getting the environment right can really help – wherever you give birth. Replicating a home-like environment, or actually giving birth at home, can give lots of us the best chance of a straightforward birth. This is borne out by evidence that women who plan home births and birth centre births, even if they end up transferring somewhere else in labour, are less likely to end up with a caesarean or instrumental birth and that women report less pain in these settings. See Chapter 11 on page 181 for more on choosing where to give birth.

But we don't all react to environments in the same way, and if you feel you will be more relaxed in hospital, want an epidural or need more medical care in your birth, you can still tweak your birth environment (wherever it is) to help your birth hormones work (see page 164).

The importance of language

While lots of chit-chat isn't generally helpful during labour, the words you do hear can be really significant. What's helpful and what hinders will be specific to you. Here are some suggestions for you to show to your birth partner. Feel free to add your own before talking them through it:

- Many labouring women don't want to chit-chat. Don't be afraid of silence unless she tells you otherwise!
- Choose positive words when you need to talk: 'She said you'd made great progress and have already started to dilate,' 'Let's try another position, as you might be more comfortable.'
- She says she can't do it? 'You are doing this, you have done a lot of it already.'
- She is afraid? 'You are safe. We are here with you.'
- She's freaking out about how long labour is going to last? Bring her back to the here and now. 'Let's just

get through the next contraction, breathe with me now, in through your nose.'

- She feels she can't cope with contractions? Offer a practical solution. 'Let's try a different position. Come with me, over here, and let's try the birth ball and I'll rub your back.' Is it time to try the shower? The birth pool? A walk? A different position? Changing the status quo can feel helpful, and it almost doesn't matter what you actually suggest doing.

- Some women need to hear loving, championing and inspirational things: 'I love you, you are so amazing and I'm really proud of you,' 'I knew you could do this. You are smashing it. Keep going.' It does sound a bit puke-worthy now, but for some women, at some points of labour, hearing the person they love affirm their confidence and support can make all the difference.

- Sometimes women in transition ask to go to hospital/to go home/to have an epidural as a way of saying that labour is suddenly overwhelming them. Focus them back on the now (and see page 128 for transition support tips). If a woman is asking for pain relief that is in her birth plan, help her get it sorted as soon as possible. If she's deviating from her plan it might just be a wobble. So suggest something in the birth plan first, or help her re-focus on her coping strategies. If she's asking repeatedly for something not in the plan, listen to her and help her get it organized. Plans can and do change.

Checklist

1. Keep doing your yoga breathing practice regularly. Try the new exercise on page 159.
2. Choose your birth goal, share it with your partner and write it down (see page 163).
3. Do the calm and stress triggers exercise (page 167), using this to help you think about where you might give birth, who you want with you and what tools and equipment you might need.
4. Make sure your partner knows how to get the most hormone-friendly set-up in your birth room (see page 164).
5. Feeling fearful? Try the exercise on page 171 to help you identify why.
6. Practise labour breathing and making funny noises. First alone and then with your partner. Try practising these while trying out the labour positions on pages 137–43.
7. Get your partner to read up on the importance of language in labour (see page 178).
8. Remember to give the tension release exercise on page 46 a try if you haven't already, and think about using this in labour.

Chapter 11

Where to Give Birth

Choosing where to have your baby can feel like the most important decision in your pregnancy. I hope that by now you've realized that the four walls around you when you give birth are only a small part of having a birth that feels right for you.

But finding a location that gives you the best chance of having the birth you want is certainly something to consider. It's also a decision that other people tend to have very strong views about. Your most useful tool for this bit may be a pair of fingers firmly jammed in your ears when your sister/mother/friend or in-law tells you what to do. Your birth, your choice, end of discussion!

I loved being at home for both my labours. Despite being a doctor's daughter and initially planning to be in hospital and have an epidural, I'd found going to hospital in pregnancy stressed me out, so I decided to avoid it if all was straightforward. For me it was great not to have to worry about when to go into hospital, or disrupt the flow of my labour with a journey. I liked using my own bath and having my possessions around me, and my husband felt more relaxed at home too. Many women I've worked with have felt happier choosing a birth centre or hospital set-up, and feel more relaxed and confident outside of the home. In this chapter we'll look at all the options, so you can make your own mind up.

The basics

Wherever you live in the UK you should be able to choose between giving birth in hospital, a birth centre within a hospital, a stand-alone birth centre, or in your own home. If you know what you want, and what the implications of that choice are in your specific circumstances, and are comfortable with those risks and benefits, you should be able to give birth in any location. In practice it can be harder to get support for a birth place of choice if you are having a more complex pregnancy and want to give birth at home or in a birth centre, or if you want to give birth by caesarean section but don't have a medical reason for this. You can get support for these choices and will find the guides to your rights and decision-making in this book particularly useful if you are in this situation.

Around the world this varies, from country to country and also from region to region. In Australia, women living in big cities should be able to choose between a hospital or birth centre birth, and many will be able to choose a home birth depending on the insurance restrictions at the time. If you live in a more remote part of Australia your options may be more limited, but you can use all the tools in the tips from the previous 2 chapters wherever you give birth.

Your midwife = your new BFF

The data doesn't lie – women who have the same midwife, or small team of midwives, caring for them in pregnancy and in birth have happier, healthier pregnancies and better births. There's a big focus on changing maternity systems to make this more common so, if you'd like to benefit from continuity of carer, ask your friends, online, your GP and your midwife to discover what's available near you.

In general you have the best chance of getting booked in with a midwife or small team who will follow you through your pregnancy if you are particularly vulnerable because of mental health issues, domestic circumstances or anxiety about the pregnancy or birth, or if you are planning a home birth.

Hospital birth

Amy had her first babies in hospital:

'When I found out I was pregnant with twins I assumed that the active birth I was hoping for would be out of the question. But we asked for a meeting with the consultant midwife and our doctor and discovered I could be active and use water as long as we understood the risks as well as the benefits. They also made it clear it was completely up to us, so we could have gone down the caesarean route if we'd wanted.

At 38 weeks my waters started leaking and after 24 hours of not much happening I had a pessary induction (see page 250 for details). By that afternoon things were moving and we went into our labour room, where we set up our aromatherapy and music. I kept active and I was dilating, but late in the night the team was concerned that it was moving much more slowly than they'd like so they

183

recommended we had a drip induction, which brings on full labour very quickly.

They explained that I could have an epidural that I could top up myself so I could decide how much pain relief I needed so I could stay mobile, so we went with this. I jacked the epidural up and rested for a few hours while the induction started working, then by the afternoon I was ready to start pushing so reduced it.

We tried a few positions and pushed for a few hours – the midwives were very encouraging, and we got to a stage where you could just feel the first baby's head, but then things stuck there and the doctors were called in. They moved us into the theatre and my heart sank slightly, but the theatre team were actually the most encouraging and inspirational bit of the whole experience. The doctors made it really clear that I was going to keep pushing the babies out, and they'd be there to help only if it was needed, which turned out to be just a very neat cut and use of a small ventouse cup (see page 240 for information on assisted births).

The midwife who'd been with us the night before came back on shift, and she led the cheerleading with Andy as I continued pushing. And then suddenly Joshua was out and immediately screaming which was the most amazing sound in the entire world. Within half an hour I was pushing again and 37 minutes after Joshua was born, Isaac came out and was just as noisy as his brother.'

The vast majority of women in the UK give birth on an obstetrician-led labour ward. On the labour ward you will have access to all the medical pain relief options, and will be close to operating theatres and neonatal support should your baby need help. The ward will be run by a consultant obstetrician, who will have a team of more junior doctors working with them. Depending on how things are going, you might not even meet a doctor but are most likely to see them during their twice-daily ward rounds. You will also have a midwife, who is the person you will spend most time with during labour, and who may actually be there to guide you through the birth.

Hospital settings are particularly good if you are having a more complicated pregnancy, are sure that you want access to an epidural, or if a hospital environment makes you feel safer and more confident. If you start in another place and develop complications you'll be offered a transfer to the labour ward. And if you decide you'd like an epidural, but are in a setting where they aren't provided, you can be transferred to the nearest labour ward to get one.

There's a current drive to encourage women to consider out-of-hospital birth settings like birth centres and home births. Coming so quickly on the tail of the drive 50 years ago to persuade women to stop giving birth at home, it's not surprising that many of us feel that hospital is the logical and safest place to give birth and feel a bit anxious about this new focus. After all, hospital is where most women currently give birth and where we are used to seeing it take place on TV.

Pros:

- You will have care from a consultant if you need one.

- No chance of needing to transfer anywhere in labour.
- You might feel more relaxed and confident in a clinical setting.
- You will have access to the full range of pain relief drugs including an epidural.
- Staff will be more accustomed to complicated pregnancies and births.

Cons:

- Significantly higher rate of unnecessary intervention.
- Women report lowest levels of satisfaction, respectful care and higher levels of pain in hospital.
- Midwife may be caring for more than one woman.
- Postnatal wards are one of the most overstretched areas in maternity care. Women sometimes have negative experiences on them.

Birth centres/midwife led units

Sarah had her first baby in a local birth centre:

 'I really enjoyed being pregnant, read as much as I could and was weirdly looking forward to the birth rather than feeling like it was an ordeal that I was dreading.

I wanted to go to the birth centre because of friends who'd had positive experiences there. This wasn't completely straightforward as I had antibodies

in my blood that could potentially harm my baby,
which meant that I was classified as 'high risk'.
Luckily my consultant was fantastic so we met with
the head midwife and it was signed off as long as
there was the right blood on standby and certain
tests were carried out on the baby.

It all kicked off one morning, a week before my
due date. It dawned on me that those stomach
cramps I'd had all morning really weren't shifting.
I lay there wondering could this be it? When
you haven't given birth before how are you meant to
know when you are in labour? But the regularity
of these pains eventually persuaded me to
call my husband Will and suggest that he might
have to come home.

I went to the toilet and there was the show,
confirming my suspicions. I giddily ran a bath
and put on some hypnobirthing scripts, dealing
with the now more frequent contractions as
best I could. The water felt good, which boded
well for the hospital pool I had been obsessing
over. Between contractions I somehow got
dressed and even put on a playlist of favourite
songs I had compiled for the birth.

Will eventually arrived home and I called him over to
push against as the contractions hit. We decided to
leave at 6 p.m. and on arrival I doubled up outside
the front of the hospital and again in the lift as
the contractions became intolerable.

We were led through to one of the birth centre rooms. A trainee male midwife took me through and could see I was in quite a lot of pain so offered me gas and air straight away. I consented to an examination which found I was already 8cm dilated. Thrilled that I hadn't arrived too early – just in the nick of time more like – and a bit high on the gas and air, I flexed my arm like a muscle emoji at Will before yelling, "Get me in that pool!" It was such a relief to be in there.

What followed is all a bit of a blur. I found it so carnal and primeval. I definitely had a wobble and said I couldn't do it but didn't ask for any other pain relief. For a change of mood I suggested that we put on the mix a DJ had played at our wedding. Will was amazing, massaging my shoulders, handing me drinks and oils, and reassuring me throughout. At one point he asked how it compared to running a marathon. "This is much worse."

Finally, less than 3 hours after we arrived at the birth centre, our baby emerged out of me into the water and was lifted out, taking its first ever breath on this planet before being placed in my arms. It took about an hour for the placenta to come out naturally and I needed a couple of stitches. I found all of this fairly unpleasant and was keen to speed things up, as I just wanted to enjoy this small creature that I was going to spend the rest of my life with. But Will encouraged me not to be the one to divert from the birth plan, for which I am very grateful.

Suddenly we were three, eating tea and toast in
bed together and discovering breastfeeding for the
first time. The birth centre was empty that night
apart from us, and so we were able to stay in the
room where Joni was born, suspending our
experience of her entry into the world for a
little longer. She and Will slept well. I could barely
close my eyes. Fundamentally changed by what
had just happened and, unknowingly so, by
what was yet to come.'

Many areas have a birth centre within the hospital and may also have separate birth centres on a different site. Birth centres are run entirely by midwives, so any more serious complications will require a transfer. They are designed to be the perfect venue to encourage your birth hormones to work (see page 164) and are designed for women having straightforward pregnancies, though some birth centres do look after women with more complex pregnancies.

Pros:

- More flexible policies on birth partners and visiting older children.
- Greater chance of a dedicated midwife.
- Lower chance of needing intervention.
- More likely to have use of birth pool.
- Better set up for active birth and often a larger, newer, nicer room.
- You may feel more relaxed and confident in a less formal setting.
- Your partner may be able to stay with you overnight after the birth. Many centres have double beds.

- Women report higher satisfaction levels, more respectful care and report lower pain in birth centres.

Cons:

- No access to epidural.
- Some areas are very strict with the criteria for birth centres, meaning it can be hard to get into one.
- Further away from the operating theatre and neonatal unit (no evidence this impacts on safety) – though some birth centres are sometimes simply at the other end of the corridor from the labour ward.

Home birth

Katie: 'We woke up on Monday morning feeling pretty resigned to the fact that I would be induced the following day at 42 weeks, but then my cramps started to become a little bit regular. We realized that they were coming around every 10 minutes. After speaking to our reassuring doula we went for a walk with our dog, stopping quite regularly for me to have another "cramp" and lean on Ollie.

When we got home the contractions were still coming regularly, but Ollie still managed to cook sausage, mash and cabbage, which we ate at the dining table with a glass of red wine.

Fairly soon we realized the contractions were coming every 5 minutes, so Ollie asked our doula to come round and notified the midwife on call.

I wasn't handling the contractions particularly well and they were making me feel a bit panicky. I found being on all fours the most comfortable position during contractions, and sat and bounced on the birthing ball between them. Our doula helped me establish a breathing pattern and noise to help cope better. Ollie helped relieve the pain of the contractions by talking me through visualizing a walk we had done in Devon on one of our favourite holidays. Step by step we walked up the hill, through the gorse, past the rocky corner up to the grassy top where we could see the sea.

The midwife arrived, unpacked and carried out some checks including my blood pressure and the baby's heartbeat, which were both fine. I wanted to get in the pool, but as I was 3cm dilated the midwife suggested we wait. I remember yelling "I can't do this" quite a few times!

At around 10 p.m. I had reached 5cm so we made the journey downstairs and I got in the pool. It was incredibly soothing to be in the water and also to be kneeling and leaning on a nice squishy surface rather than the carpet or bed cover. After lots of extremely fierce contractions where I was feeling the urge to push quite strongly, the midwife asked me to get out

to be examined again. I was fully dilated after less
than 2 hours in the pool.

I got back on all fours on the living-room rug.
I tried sitting on a bucket which really helped the
baby come down but intensified the pain.
Somewhere in my mind I recognized that
gravity was really going to help me out, so I
actually got up from the bucket and stood
upright. Ollie sat on the sofa and I leaned
on his thighs. With each contraction, I
squatted a little bit.

We managed to see the baby's head in a mirror.
What an extraordinary sight! It helped me focus
though, and with the next contraction, he was
passed between my legs.'

Different areas run home birth services in different ways.
Some rely on a large team of community midwives on a rota
to attend to women in labour at home. Others have a smaller,
dedicated home birth team, giving you a good chance of seeing the same midwife throughout pregnancy and having her
(or one of her colleagues who you may well have met) for
your labour.

Pros:

- No restrictions on partners or visiting hours.
- You have 2 midwives dedicated to you.
- Only 10 per cent chance of needing intervention.
- Guaranteed use of birth pool.

- You and your partner may feel more relaxed and confident in your own home.
- All the comforts of home, and you can be tucked up in your own bed afterwards and eat whatever you like.
- Women report highest satisfaction levels, most respectful care and report lower pain at home.

Cons:

- No access to epidural or pethidine.
- Some areas have a patchy service and you might have to go in to hospital on the day.
- Further away from operating theatre and neonatal care (though evidence suggests this doesn't impact on safety).
- Some women feel safer in hospital.

The evidence about interventions and safety

In England we have some really high-quality evidence on the safety of different birth settings, and, though set-ups are slightly different across the UK, it's a useful guide wherever you live. The Birthplace in England study (2011) looked at 70,000 low-risk women who gave birth. It was conducted by Oxford University and is one of the biggest and most robust studies on the topic ever done. Here are the results:

- Between 4 and 5 in every 10 women who started their labour in a hospital labour ward ended up with a significant intervention such as an assisted birth or a caesarean (see pages 240 and 232).

- For women who planned to use a birth centre, that rate of intervention dramatically dropped to around 2 in every 10 women.
- One woman out of every 10 who planned a home birth ended up with a significant intervention (after a transfer to hospital).

Based on this evidence, women having straightforward pregnancies and those keen to avoid intervention unless it is necessary are often advised to consider giving birth away from a hospital.

This study also looked at the safety of the baby in each setting. **For all babies, wherever they were born, birth in England was found to be very safe.** Rates of stillbirth and very serious injury were so low that the researchers decided to look at a wider category of 'serious outcomes'. These included serious and tragic events such as stillbirth or death of the baby, potentially life-threatening complications resulting in long-term disability, and less severe conditions which may require treatment (perhaps in a neonatal unit) but which may not necessarily result in any long-term problems for the baby. Collectively, and on average, only 4 babies in every 1,000 births had one of these complications.

For second-time, or more, mothers, labour ward, birth centre and home birth were found to be almost identical in terms of safety.

For first-time mothers, the baby was equally safe in all settings apart from a small increase in the risk of a serious poor outcome at home births. That increased risk is equivalent to 4 additional babies in every 1,000 having a serious outcome among first-time mothers who plan a home birth.

Elective caesarean sections

Charlotte had her third baby via a 'skin-to-skin' caesarean section – also called a 'natural caesarean' or 'family-centred caesarean'. The procedure isn't widely available on the NHS, though elements of it may be able to be replicated if you talk to your obstetrician in advance. Any baby born by caesarean section, and who doesn't need immediate help from the paediatric team, should have immediate skin-to-skin if you want to.

> ❝ 'I'd had my first 2 children at this hospital by C-section and had often wondered what it would be like to actually hold your baby before it is whisked off to be weighed. While I was eternally grateful for 2 healthy

195

children who may well never have made it into this world without the grace of medical advances, I still wondered about it. So I was really interested in taking part in a trial of 'skin-to-skin' caesareans happening at the hospital.

The atmosphere in theatre was one of eager anticipation, and despite the familiar array of catheters, scalpels and needles to administer the spinal epidural, I found myself grinning with excitement. My husband is next to me and all goes according to plan. The spinal being administered is a bit nerve-racking but not exactly painful and then it takes about 5 minutes of really bizarre-feeling rummaging until my son's head and then body slowly starts to emerge. He pushes and squeezes his way out into the world, clearing his own lungs, as he would have done during a vaginal birth.

Then, once the screen between us has been lowered, he is placed on my chest with his cord still attached – still covered in mucus. While my other children had screamed for minutes on end after first emerging, he immediately calms.

As a mother of 3 I've been buoyed by the memory of watching my child emerge, triumphantly, into the theatre like a small, warm and very hairy statue of liberty. Not to mention the sense of fulfilment at being the first one to welcome him, soothe and protect him from the throbbing noise and bright lights of the outside world.'

"

Around a quarter of births now happen by caesarean section in the UK and rates have been steadily rising over the past few decades. For some women, the level of control and ability to plan their baby's birth that a caesarean section offers means that they are keen to have this option whether or not there is a medical reason.

Caesarean risks and benefits

Giving birth by caesarean involves a different set of benefits and risks to giving birth vaginally. These will differ from woman to woman and from pregnancy to pregnancy. Overall, planned caesarean section has been found to be safer for woman and baby than emergency caesarean. However, all caesareans are considered to be a very safe intervention, and the risks of serious outcomes are small. Your midwife and doctor should talk you through the pros and cons in your situation and share the evidence that these are based on. To find out more, read the NICE guidelines on caesarean sections: www.nice.org.uk/guidance/cg132.

If you are thinking that you would like to have a caesarean section, and you do not have a particular medical indication, it's worth reading Chapter 5 to learn more about your rights. If there are no medical reasons, you do not have a specific legal guarantee of being able to choose a caesarean on the NHS, but best practice guidelines mean that, after jumping through a couple of hoops, your request should be granted. Some women find the process of getting a caesarean section approved completely draining, and some NHS Trusts have stricter policies than others. Private obstetricians may be able to offer maternal request caesareans more easily.

Lisa had already had a traumatic miscarriage. Both her sisters and her mother had ended up with emergency caesarean sections (see page 232).

> **"** 'I felt really anxious about the thought of giving birth. Just felt like I couldn't do it. I'd really hated how much people had fiddled with me when I needed to concentrate during my miscarriage. I felt like I'd rather just know what was happening from the beginning. I met with the consultant midwife to talk about it and she let me know that as well as a caesarean I could give birth at home, or in the midwife-led unit in the birth pool. I didn't have to have any examinations, I didn't have to have any injections or needles and we could just take it at my pace. I decided on the birth centre but we also agreed that if anything went wrong, I needed an induction or there was slow progress we would just go straight for a caesarean.' **"**

Being able to control the birth plan and discuss her fears really helped Lisa, even though she ended up having an emergency caesarean section.

> **"** 'I actually really loved my labour. I think that knowing I had the bail-out option just made me more relaxed. I spent ages at home with my boyfriend and it was quite a laugh despite the contractions. The time we spent at the birth centre

was great, the midwife was lovely and I got to use the pool. I have really positive memories of it and I feel really proud of how well I coped. Just before I was fully dilated my waters broke and there was loads of meconium (see page 246) in them. I just knew it was game over then, but they were really respectful and let me make the decision. Though it was an emergency caesarean, the baby wasn't in distress and I was fine so we had loads of time. They knew how important skin-to-skin contact was for me, and so we had that in theatre. I'm really pleased that I asked for the elective caesarean because otherwise I wouldn't have got to meet the consultant midwife who helped with the planning.' **"**

Checklist

1. Visit the Which? Birth Choices website to find out what options are available near you.
2. Talk to your partner about your options and preferences.
3. Find out from your midwife if there are any particular birth place recommendations in your situation.
4. Use the BRAIN tool (see page 223) and the advice in Chapter 5, 'Your Rights', if you think you may want to choose an option that isn't being recommended.

Chapter 12

Overcoming a Difficult Birth

If you've had a traumatic, difficult or upsetting birth in the past, I know that pregnancy and facing the prospect of labour and birth again can bring those feelings to the front of your mind. It can make seemingly simple decisions about this next birth feel mountainous, and just being pregnant again can trigger frightening memories from your last birth. If this is ringing bells with you, let me reassure you that it's a totally normal reaction to being pregnant. I've worked with lots of women who've felt like this, and it's a completely understandable reaction to a trauma that you don't need to feel ashamed of. And despite that, you can go on to have a resoundingly different and better experience in this new pregnancy.

You are in a really strong position – much stronger than when you had your last baby – to help yourself and those caring for you make this birth the one you need. Why?

- You can learn from your last birth, discover what went well and what didn't, and shape a better birth plan.
- You've likely experienced at least part of labour before. It's not the unknown any more, and you will have a sense of how you coped with contractions and what other tools you need to work on.

- You'll know what you need in a partner and who or what isn't helpful.
- Your body is on your side. If you've laboured before (even if you didn't dilate all the way last time), and especially if you've given birth vaginally, this labour is likely to be shorter. The average second labour is 3 hours shorter than the average first.

The basics

If you have had a previously traumatic birth, you may wish to start by working out whether you need professional support through this pregnancy. If you have previously been diagnosed with post-traumatic stress disorder (PTSD), have sought counselling because of a previous birth, or are experiencing regular nightmares, flashbacks or panic attacks, then you might benefit from some expert help through this pregnancy. Your midwife or GP might be a good first port of call, and do check out www.rebeccaschiller.co.uk/noguilt for private options and supportive websites, twitter groups and forums. Eye movement desensitization and reprocessing therapy has been shown to have really good results with this kind of trauma. A detraumatizing technique called 'rewind' has also been used successfully with women who have birth trauma.

If you feel able to manage this without outside help, I've included some suggestions, based on my experience of working with many women and families following a difficult birth. It's a topic I've written about in journals and spoken about at conferences, but – spoiler alert – I am not a medical professional, a psychiatrist or psychologist. And while I've roped some of my expert clinical friends in to help, this isn't intended to replace professional help if you need it.

" Amelia: 'We'd been trying for nearly a year and really wanted another baby. I thought I was over my son's birth. I'd loved being a mother to him and had waited 3 years until I felt totally ready to do it again. But the moment I realized I was pregnant I started having feelings of anxiety about the birth and having flashbacks to last time. A lot of my early excitement was just trampled over by worry.'

Amrita: 'I was planning everything down to the finest detail. I did enough research for a thesis, bought so many different products designed to give me the best pregnancy and birth. I joined every forum, chat group, followed a million different blogs. I think I was using it to distract myself from the basics of simply coming to terms with what happened before and how I was going to handle it this time.' "

Getting information

It can be really helpful to start by understanding what happened during your last birth. Getting hold of the notes from your previous labour can be really useful, and you have a right to access these and read them without charge. Ask your midwife or call your maternity unit to arrange to see your notes. If you'd like a copy posted to you there may be a fee.

All maternity units should run a clinic, or service (sometimes called 'birth reflections' or 'birth afterthoughts'), where a senior midwife or doctor will go through your previous notes with you, giving you the chance to ask questions and get a better understanding of what happened last time. It can also be a good time to begin to talk about your options for this birth, but only if you feel ready.

If you and your partner have avoided talking much about the birth since it happened, it can feel increasingly like the elephant in the room. You may want to warn them that you would like to have a conversation about it in advance and give them time to get used to the idea. Partners can also be traumatized by difficult birth experiences, so they may wish to read the notes separately or with you and you could discuss whether it would be helpful for them to attend any appointments.

Processing your last birth

If you have had or have PTSD or think you may have some of the symptoms mentioned above (flashbacks, panic attacks, re-playing the birth over and over again), then it's crucial that you seek medical support before working out if and how to process your last birth. The exercises below might not be appropriate for you, as talking about the traumatic event in detail can sometimes re-traumatize you and make you feel worse rather than better. However, for many women who don't have PTSD, but still feel distressed by their last birth, doing some work to understand and come to terms with what happened and why can be really helpful. If you don't know which group you fall into it's worth seeking professional support. Go to www.rebeccaschiller.co.uk/noguilt for more details of how to find some.

Over a period of weeks or months (take it at your own pace) you could:

- Write down the story of your previous birth and encourage your partner to do the same.
- If you don't feel able to write it down, consider talking it through with your doula, midwife or a friend. Your partner may well remember things differently. This is totally normal and OK – both recollections are real.
- Use the birth art exercise below to consider what happened.

Exercise: Birth art

Using art to process experiences and emotion has been shown to help us increase our understanding of an event, regulate our emotions, accept and integrate an experience and change our perceptions and behaviours.

Find yourself some large sheets of paper and ideally some pastels. Failing that any old crayons or felt tips will do. Do you feel comfortable drawing the key moments of your last birth? If so, try choosing 1 from the beginning, 1 from the end and 2 from the middle that stand out for you for any reason. You can do this even if you are rubbish at drawing – stick figures work fine!

AND/OR choose the 3 most positive moments from that birth. Three things you remember that were OK for you or even felt good. Perhaps the excitement of the beginning, or when you held your baby for the first time? It could be the memory of a kind midwife or anaesthetist? Then draw the 3 most difficult moments too.

It would be really helpful for your partner to do this exercise too. You can discuss whether you are happy to see each other's and discuss them.

When you are ready, look back on your drawings and/or your writing. Use them to try to understand the good parts of your last birth. What needs of yours were being met? Was it that you felt listened to? Or that you were in charge? That you were coping with the contractions? Or didn't feel alone? This will help you ensure that you know what's important to you and can plan for your needs to be met during this birth.

Then think about the difficult stuff. Why were those moments so bad? Was it because you were frightened? Because you didn't know what was going on? Was somebody unkind to you? Did you feel like no one was helping you? Were you afraid something bad was happening to you and your baby? Now you know what you, your birth partner and your team can work on minimizing this time.

Moving on

With a handle on the ups and downs of last time, you can now make a new plan for this new birth. Start with that list of positives and negatives and use them to inform your calm and stress triggers, using the exercise on page 167.

You'll now have a concrete list, informed by you, your life

and your last birth, of what you need to turn up and turn down for this birth. Take these as your guide as you work through the birth plan in Chapter 21.

Once you have a plan that you are beginning to be happy with, you might want to meet with the head of midwifery at your maternity unit, or a consultant midwife. The midwife you met at your birth afterthoughts appointment is often a good person to start with. You can use this appointment to go through your plan, cover anything you haven't considered and discuss any requests that aren't completely standard. Having had some previously difficult times can make you understandably more particular. If you found vaginal examinations problematic last time, you may wish to avoid them. You may have ended up with a more complicated birth, but only feel confident having a home birth this time. Or know you need to request a caesarean even though you don't have any classic medical indications.

Your midwife or doctor should help you get what you need. But don't wait until 39 weeks or labour itself to ask. Have the conversation in advance and get it documented in your notes, so that you can get on with your birth without too many interruptions when the day comes and whoever looks after you on the day will feel more confident.

Where to give birth

Amrita's story: 'I'm not going to bore you with the details of my first birth. But it was long and I wasn't treated very well. After going into crazy-planning mode in my second pregnancy I landed upon hiring a doula – another impulse purchase – but thank god I did. She calmed me down about 200 per cent and got me talking to my partner, my midwife and going through my notes rather than just buying stuff I couldn't afford.

I'd gone through about 10 different birth plans: home birth, freebirth, early epidural, birth centre, and I just couldn't settle with any of them. They all made me feel worried. Then my obstetrician laid out all the options again and mentioned someone who had requested a caesarean in a similar situation. It was a lightbulb moment and I instantly felt happier. The caesarean wasn't a walk in the park, and recovery with my 2-year-old bouncing around wasn't straightforward, but it was overwhelmingly a good experience. Calm, happy, and I felt I'd made the right decision.'

"

Logistics

If you didn't have a great birth at hospital X, or with midwife Y, you might find you'd like to make sure you are in a different place this time. You are absolutely entitled to self-refer to a different hospital. You do not have to give birth at the most local location. Your GP may also be able to refer you directly to the place you would prefer to be.

Getting to know a midwife or a small midwifery team might help you feel more cared for and trusting. See page 182 for more on what might be available. Women who've had traumatic births within the NHS have often turned to independent midwives for future pregnancies. Currently, many of these private midwives are unable to practise because of insurance issues. However, there are schemes available, some of them funded by the NHS, that enable some areas to have access to independent midwife style care. See www.rebeccaschiller. co.uk/noguilt for more information.

Vaginal birth after caesarean (VBAC)

If you had a previous caesarean you should be offered the option to have a vaginal birth or another caesarean in this new pregnancy. Depending on the reasons for your first caesarean, how this pregnancy is going and how you felt about your first birth, you may already feel very strongly about how you would like to give birth this time.

VBACs are generally considered very safe. The main risk is of your previous caesarean scar rupturing during labour. This happens to around 1 in 300 women and your team will be looking for any warning signs of this, such as bleeding or pain between contractions.

Between 7 and 9 in 10 women who plan a VBAC do have a vaginal birth. If you've had 2 or 3 previous caesareans, your risks and chances of having a VBAC are about the same as if you'd had one caesarean.

If you are thinking about whether or not to plan a VBAC, you might find your hospital's VBAC clinic a useful source of information. These clinics are often run by midwives who are able to talk you through your last birth and help you come up with a tailored plan for this time.

There are some standard protocols that many hospitals encourage you to have if you are having a VBAC. These include giving birth on the labour ward, having a cannula inserted during labour just in case, and being continuously monitored. Your team can explain to you the risks and benefits of each of these suggestions for your particular situation. Some women feel these protocols might inhibit their chances of labouring well and choose to decline some or all of them. You'll want to do your own research, and there are suggestions on www.rebeccaschiller.co.uk/noguilt.

> **Cait: 'I was happy to have extra monitoring. I felt like things could go wrong quickly and, though it was smooth sailing this time, the vigilance was like a comfort blanket.'**
>
> **Amanda: 'I felt that all the fiddling about in my first birth had led to the caesarean and that I needed to maximize my chances of it going right. I negotiated that I would use the birth centre (after 40 minutes on the monitor on arrival), would have a water birth and wouldn't have a cannula unless it was actually needed.'**

Speak to your team about whether they have a birth pool on the labour ward, and a wireless, waterproof monitor if you'd like to use water but aren't sure about being in a midwife-led setting.

Michelle had two caesareans, followed by a hospital VBAC and then a home water birth. She employed an independent midwife (who works privately, not within the NHS) to care for her in her final pregnancy.

" Michelle: 'I chose home birth because I knew this was going to be my last birth. I had spent the last 3 years since my previous hospital VBAC researching and gaining as much knowledge about birth as I could. I didn't fear birth but I did fear surgery. I knew that this time I didn't want to be observed and have numerous strangers entering my birth space. When my midwife Kay said she didn't intend to treat me any differently to any other woman she had cared for, I could have cried. It was truly wonderful to end my birthing days with the most beautiful, empowering birth. It was instinctive, intimate, undisturbed, empowering, peaceful, and I was in control at every moment.' **"**

Checklist

1. Think about whether you need professional support and, if so, go to www.rebeccaschiller.co.uk/noguilt to explore your options.
2. Get hold of your previous maternity notes and make an appointment with the birth afterthoughts service (see page 202).
3. Choose an exercise from pages 204–5 to help you process your last birth. Feel free to do more than one.
4. Work the learning from this exercise into your calm and stress triggers (page 167) and use it to inform your birth plan (page 344).
5. Arrange to meet with a senior midwife, to ensure they understand your birth plan and can help you minimize any trauma triggers in this birth.

Chapter 13

Your Decisions

I'm big on decision-making, and while making decisions in labour definitely needs some thought and preparation, there's no reason why you can't be in control of what happens to your birth, body and baby.

Before labour

While you can't know what exactly is going to happen when you give birth, it's definitely worth researching the different options available to you, making any choices you can well in advance and writing a birth plan. Some decisions you can make ahead of labour include:

Birth partners

My husband was a brilliant birth partner. I wasn't sure he was going to be, but he was calm, cheerful and unflappable. He did what I asked without much question, managed the logistics pretty well, stayed quiet and out of my way apart from when I needed him, and didn't panic when our second baby was born before our midwife arrived.

I've seen some incredible husbands, sisters, friends and

girlfriends supporting women through labour. But not everyone is cut out to be the ultimate birth partner.

> **"** Susie: 'Let's just put it this way, if I have another baby I don't want my husband there and he doesn't want to be there either. We both think it's a mistake them being there at all and can't work out why it took me THREE births to realize it didn't work. I wish I'd paid for a doula.' **"**

Giving birth is one thing that most of us don't want to do alone. There's plenty of evidence that, for the overwhelming majority of women, having the right person supporting you through birth can improve how you feel about it and also make labour itself easier and more straightforward.

Choosing a birth partner

I can't tell you who will be the right helper to have by your side. But here are a few suggestions that may help you make your decision.

Think about your list of calm and stress triggers (see page 167). No one who ticks more stress than calm boxes should be in your labour room. Most women choose their partners in life as their partners in birth. This can be wonderful. Your partner is often the person who knows you best and should be able to de-stress and relax you quickly. But not all girlfriends/boyfriends/husbands or wives make great birth partners. If in times of stress your partner drives you mad, if they are very squeamish or just don't actually want to be there, you might need to have an open conversation with them to discover

---

whether they might be better left at home with a list of things to clean. Mothers or sisters can provide amazing support, but think carefully if they've had difficult births themselves and might bring their anxiety into your birth room.

Doulas can be the ultimate birth supporters. They can provide respite, pressure-relieving and guidance to your partner (but never replace them), experienced, hands-on and emotional support through pregnancy, labour itself and the first weeks with your new baby. Studies have shown that women who have continuous support in labour have happier, faster labours, request less pain relief, have less intervention and their babies are born in better condition. These effects are most dramatic when the supporter isn't a family member, friend or a member of hospital staff.

Exercise: What I need from you

Sit down with your birth partners. Talk about what you need from each other during labour and birth. Consider how you want them to speak to you, how you want decisions to be handled, what you want them to avoid doing, explain any pet hates and any definite needs. Ask them to feel able to tell you what they need from you.

Examples:

'I need you to speak to me quietly and calmly, especially in a stressful situation.' 'I need you to tell me what is happening.' 'If you are feeling stressed I need you to go for a walk, talk to your friend, and come back feeling calmer.' 'I need you to practise massaging me so that you can do so without pummelling me.' 'I need you to keep your mother out of the picture.' 'I need you to get off your phone during labour.' 'I need you to eat, take naps, and look after yourself too.'

Vaginal examinations

If you choose to have vaginal examinations (VEs), your midwife or doctor will ask for your consent before inserting 2 fingers into your vagina and then into your cervix. They will move their fingers apart to estimate how open it is, how much of the cervix they can still feel and also what position your baby is in. You will be offered these routinely every 4 hours and may also be offered one if your team need to know where your labour is at, right at that moment before making a decision about whether to intervene or not.

VEs can be a useful baseline for you and your caregivers, particularly when making these decisions about interventions. Some women like to have a reassuring snapshot of how their labour is going, but in a straightforward labour VEs' usefulness is limited. Women can find them uncomfortable or painful, it can be difficult to get into the right position for them when contractions are coming regularly, and they can give you and your team a distorted picture of what's happening in labour. Just because your cervix isn't very open right now doesn't mean that a strong labour won't open it all the way very soon. Women can and often do have a non-linear pattern to dilation. Like with any procedure, you can decline routine vaginal examinations.

Monitoring

In a straightforward birth your midwife will assess how well your baby is coping with labour by listening in to their heart rate every 15 minutes using a handheld doppler monitor – the same kind they use at your antenatal appointments. During the second stage of labour they will offer to listen in to the baby more often – every 5 minutes, often after a contraction.

You can decline all or some of this monitoring, or request an extra 'listen in' if it would help set your mind at rest. Midwives will try to hear your baby's heartbeat in the position you are already in, but may ask you to change position if they are having difficulty picking it up.

If you are having a more complex pregnancy, or are giving birth on the labour ward, or have an epidural sited, your midwife or doctor will probably recommend that you have continuous foetal monitoring. If you agree, then two soft, stretchy belts are put around your belly. One will monitor your baby's heart rate and the other your contractions. These are recorded continuously by a nearby machine.

This kind of monitoring is not recommended if you are having a low-risk pregnancy, as it has been shown to have no benefit for you or your baby, yet dramatically increases your risk of having an unnecessary intervention.

If you have a more complicated pregnancy you will want to find out what benefit continuous monitoring will offer in your specific situation and understand any associated risks. Continuous monitoring can make being active and getting comfortable in different positions really difficult, but wireless monitors are often available, so do ask to use one if moving around is important to you. Wireless monitors are often waterproof, meaning that labouring or giving birth in water is still on the cards even if you want to be continuously monitored.

Episiotomy or tearing naturally

In the UK around 19 out of 100 women have an episiotomy – a cut that is made in the perineum to widen the opening and allow the baby to be born, with numbers being significantly higher if this is a first baby. Episiotomies are offered to speed up the birth process in an emergency situation, in the rare cases when the perineum is not stretching around the baby's head after a long time pushing, or to facilitate an assisted birth.

Practice differs around the world, but the evidence clearly demonstrates that, in most situations, it is far better to have a natural tear, which will heal faster, be less likely to become infected and cause less pain. You are only likely to be offered an episiotomy in very specific circumstances and you can use a decision-making tool (the BRAIN tool, explained in detail on page 223) to help work out what's right for you. Do remember that, as with any intervention, it is always your right to decline.

Third stage of labour

After pushing an entire human being out of your vagina you should get let off hard work for a bit. But after any vaginal birth you will need to give birth to your placenta – the incredible, albeit slightly gory, organ that has been keeping your baby alive for 9 months. There are decisions to make around how you would like the third stage to be managed and when you would like to clamp and cut the cord. There are benefits and risks to all the different options, which will change depending on your circumstances. Think through these in advance, as you will be far more interested in your new baby at the time. If your situation changes in labour, your midwife will offer to change this part of your birth in response.

Active management of the third stage

If you opt for this you'll be given an injection of syntocinon or Syntometrine in your thigh as or soon after your baby is born. The injection mimics and accelerates the body's own processes and is designed to minimize bleeding and get the placenta out quickly. It's particularly suitable for women at higher risk of bleeding or who have had intervention in their labour. Within 5 minutes your midwife will check progress by feeling your abdomen and gently pulling on the cord. You may push the placenta out or they might help you by controlled pulling on the cord. Traditionally the cord is clamped and cut straight away, but increasingly best practice is to leave it for between 1 and 5 minutes during active management.

Advantages:

- Placenta born faster.
- Less blood loss, though if you are at low risk of bleeding heavily this won't be significant.
- Lessens your risk of haemorrhage after birth if you are at medium or high risk of losing too much blood, for example, after a forceps birth or if you are anaemic.

Disadvantages:

- A significant minority of women feel sick, dizzy or faint after the injection.
- Can alter your blood pressure.
- Lower birth weight of baby (as often associated with early cord clamping).
- You are more likely to return to hospital with abnormal bleeding after you've been discharged.

> **Soraya: 'I didn't really know I had a choice to opt for a managed third stage first time around and so I found myself having the injection. It didn't hurt and it meant that the placenta business was over and done with really quickly and I could focus on having time with my baby, so I was keen to do it again. I did want to leave the cord to pulsate for a bit second time around and so I negotiated with my midwife that they would leave it for a couple of minutes before clamping and cutting.'**

Physiological third stage

Having a physiological third stage means relying on your body's own processes to manage blood loss, expel the placenta and contract the uterus. It's ideal if you've had a straightforward birth without any intervention and aren't at risk of bleeding heavily. If you opt for this method, your midwife will still have the injection to hand in case you do start to bleed too much after birth.

Advantages:

- No reaction to the synthetic hormones such as sickness or blood pressure changes.
- Timing of cord clamping is more flexible.
- Less likely to have problems later on with bleeding.
- Less interruption during first 10 minutes (or longer) with baby.

Disadvantages:

- Losing more blood (though only 80ml on average).
- If you are at medium/high risk of haemorrhage your risk of this increases significantly.
- Takes on average 10 minutes longer for the placenta to be born.
- You may need to work a bit harder to birth it, though this shouldn't be painful.

> Natalie: 'When my twins were born they were whisked off, checked and wrapped up. It felt like ages before I held them and it took me quite a while to understand and believe that they were mine. With my next child I was determined it would be different. I didn't want the injection for the placenta and I wanted to leave the cord intact until after the placenta was born. Partly to get as much blood into my baby as possible but I also really liked the idea of having a physical connection between us for that first hour or so. So we'd already had a good cuddle and a feed by the time that my placenta was born.'

If you are having a physiological third stage, best practice guidelines state that if your placenta isn't born within about an hour of your baby you should be offered active management.

> If you are opting for a physiological third stage, remember that your hormones still need to do their thing – just like in labour. You'll be helped by a dark, quiet, calm and loving environment. Holding, breastfeeding and doing skin-to-skin with your baby will help the placenta be born. If your placenta is taking a while, make sure you aren't getting cold or hungry, and try sitting on a birth stool or bucket.

Cord clamping

New evidence has emerged, and guidelines on cord clamping and cutting have changed. It's now recommended that all babies' cords are left to pulsate for at least 1 minute after birth, unless they have partially snapped during the birth or the baby needs resuscitating and they don't have facilities to do this at the bedside.

Why? Studies have shown that one third of a baby's blood volume stays in the placenta after birth and that clamping the cord too soon deprives them of blood they need. Babies who are allowed to benefit from this can have a wide range of better health outcomes, including better iron levels and stores up to 6 months of age. It can be particularly good for babies born prematurely and for unwell newborns.

If the cord clamping is delayed there is a small increase in the number of babies who develop jaundice (from 3 in 100 in the immediately clamped group to 5 in 100 in the delayed clamping group).

Decision-making in labour

Research shows that feeling in control, well supported and informed is crucial to feeling good about your baby's birth. For this to happen it helps if you know how to get and synthesize good, accurate and complete information from those who are caring for you.

> Emily: 'After an induction to start my first labour I wanted as few interventions as possible in my second. But after a night at the birth centre in strong labour, daylight started to break and my labour slowed. The midwife suggested transferring to hospital and having a hormone drip. My knee-jerk reaction was both "Oh no" and "Oh yes". I knew I hated that drip from last time but I was also really tempted by the thought of an epidural, a rest and getting things over with sooner rather than later.
>
> My husband encouraged me to take some time to think about it, got me comfortable, found some food and drink and took the pressure off. We realized we had questions we hadn't asked, so asked the midwife to come back and we talked through everything. We found out what the risks were and how we'd deal with them. How we'd know if the baby and I were still OK and what the problems carrying on in the birth centre might be. Then we talked about what the transfer would be like if we went for that.

We came to the conclusion that I was really
exhausted and I just needed a rest. We
agreed we wouldn't have more vaginal examinations
during the day but I would do a mixture of
walking and resting.

As soon as darkness fell again my contractions
ramped back up. I was really determined that
this was it now, so I was back in the room
using all the different positions the midwife
could suggest to get things going. It soon became
very clear that this was not stopping. Suddenly
I was pushing and shortly after I was holding the
baby. I'm so glad that we didn't just say yes to
the first option but worked out what we needed
for ourselves. And if I'd had to transfer later on
I think I would've been happier at least
knowing I'd given it a good shot.'

"

Checklist

1. Think carefully about birth partners and consider
   hiring a doula (page 212).
2. Work through the 'What I need from you' exercise
   with your birth partner (see page 213).
3. Decide what monitoring you would prefer and
   discuss what is recommended for you with your
   midwife (see page 215).
4. Discuss routine vaginal examinations (see page 214)
   with your midwife.
5. Practise the BRAIN technique (on the following
   page) for decision-making with your partner.

BRAIN

It can be hard to remember what questions to ask when you are busy labouring, so get your partner to memorize this acronym: BRAIN. I can't claim credit for it myself – and I'm not sure anyone knows where it originated – but I've used it loads of times to great effect.

B = Benefits. What is the benefit of a specific course of action? Make sure these benefits are specific to you.

R = Risk. What are the risks of this specific course of action? Again, make sure these are specific to you.

A = Alternatives. As in Emily's birth, are there any alternatives available? Can you think of any yourselves and test them out with your team?

I = Instincts. What is your gut feeling about this?

N = Nothing. What happens if you do nothing? If the answer is simply (as it often is) that you'll continue to wait, check that you and the baby remain fine and wait for the baby to be born or something to change, this gives you a really good way to gauge the urgency of the situation.

Chapter 14

The Unexpected

If you haven't had a baby before, then you might find some of the things your body does, the ways you behave in labour or how you feel, are a surprise or a shock. Even if you're an old hand at birthing, second and third labours have a funny old habit of being different to those before.

My first labour started with my waters breaking mid-afternoon. At 11 p.m. I went into labour and before 7 a.m. the next morning I was holding my daughter. When my waters broke mid-afternoon kicking off my second birth I imagined that, once again, I'd be holding a baby by breakfast – if not before. Much to my extreme annoyance this second time, my labour didn't start in earnest until the following lunchtime and then unfolded at breakneck speed in 40 minutes. Everything felt different at that speed.

What was the most unexpected thing about your labour and birth?

 Claire: 'That my husband would be so panicked when we drove to hospital for baby number one that he'd crash the car into a lamppost in the car park.'

Michelle: 'How important my intuition was, how powerful it was to really rely on myself and how incredible my body and mind are.'

Amy: 'It was definitely the feeling of my section. It was the oddest sensation to be in no pain, yet feel every rummage as my twins were pulled out. I wasn't expecting the sheer brute force of the tugging!'

Holly: 'That due dates have "estimated" in front of them for a reason. And some of them are total bollocks. I knew my cycles and when I'd conceived so was certain my dates were putting me a week ahead. I insisted we go by my dates, not the scan dates as I didn't want to be pressurized into an induction before my baby was ready to be born.'

Clara: 'That my breasts would be bigger than my baby's head. Shocking!'

Lisa: 'That it was totally doable once I learnt how and I didn't need the caesarean I thought I wanted.'

Claire: 'That everyone else seemed to be wafting into the maternity ward, whereas I was on all fours, screaming and already 8cm dilated. It was a quick but intense labour . . . ouch.'

Jacqui: 'The mucus plug! I was expecting something akin to an earplug or bath-plug so was quite shocked when the hand-sized blood-streaked pile of slime oozed out on to the floor!'

Catherine: 'That I'd poo during labour. I've had 4 babies and pooed every time. The first time I was so shocked and embarrassed but now I know that it is just a totally normal part of pushing a baby out.'

Kay: 'That I wouldn't poo when I gave birth. All my friends warned me about it and it used to petrify me. But as soon as contractions started I was on the loo with an upset tummy, so there was nothing left to come out!'

Fiona: 'How different one birth can be from the last one – and how much of that is down to your midwife. I'd had a horrible first birth but I had a midwife I knew second time around and I trusted her implicitly. All my scepticism and raised eyebrows about birth not being awful went out the window.'

Natalie: 'That if they say it's going to be a quick birth, you should listen to them. It'll save you from having your large, stretch-marked bum in the air giving birth in a car outside the hospital. The round of applause was just a little embarrassing realizing everyone had seen.'

Kate: 'How long my labour would be. On and off for a few days before it really got going and about 3 days in hospital, gradually being induced more and more until an eventual caesarean. It felt like I'd entered another space/time dimension.'

Anna: 'The shock of the power of the contractions and what my body can do.'

Catherine: 'That when it sounds like an animal has entered the room, those noises are you and you've almost got your baby.'

Becky: 'That birth can be an amazing experience. Sure it is painful, but it is so much more than that too.'

Maisie: 'The way gas and air makes me feel. I was totally high, saying really inappropriate stuff to the very young midwife and cracking crazy jokes. Pretty sure I was hallucinating at one point too. I fucking loved it.'

Jacqui: 'That I'd make the weirdest noises in labour. I suddenly said, "Oh my god, it sounds like I'm having really good sex," a thought which made me promptly throw up!'

Isabel: 'That, though everyone says waters breaking isn't like in the movies, mine was a spectacular cinematic gush, all over the floor of the lift at the hospital. Sorry fellow lift-riders.'

Anna: 'The sheer exhilaration of meeting your baby, whatever the method of birth or pain relief you've had.'

Lyndsey: 'How good it felt to push! It was my favourite part of both my labours.'

Jay: 'That I would want to marry the anaesthetist who gave me the epidural and told him that I loved him about twenty times.'

Amy: 'That I wouldn't really notice transition, or make loud noises. I was very quiet and inside myself – it helped me cope. Not like me at all – you usually can't shut me up.'

Anna: 'Giving birth is my favourite part of the whole thing. Hate pregnancy. Not wild about the early days with the baby (though I like them when they start smiling) but I really, really loved giving birth. It was really hard and easy all at the same time and, especially as things haven't always gone smoothly, when I'm having a tough time in life I look back on those births and I think I can do anything.'

"

Complex births

"

Emily: 'I had created an ideal birth plan, which included no pain relief, little to no monitoring, birth centre, exclusively breastfeeding and getting home as quickly as possible after birth. But I developed pre-eclampsia and I was induced, monitored like a lab rat and gave birth in an obstetric unit. He went to the special care baby unit and was fed by drip, then donor breast milk, any drops of milk I could get from expressing and mainly formula.

Given all this you would think I had the worst birth ever, but actually it was wonderful. Writing the birth plan was key – even though it changed. It was incredible how much time our midwife spent reading it and ensuring that she could do everything possible to make our birth as much like it as she could. She respected our wishes, trusted me and my body, monitored me discreetly and was very hands off.

Even though we had our birth plan organized to every last detail we were always pragmatic. Complications can happen in childbirth, which we acknowledged when writing our birth plan. My husband and I agreed together that we would try hard to trust the staff at our hospital to hear our voices and let them help us make the best decision we could.

This may sound strange having just said "trust your team", but I also learned from my experience that a skilled maternity team knows to trust a woman and what she says about her body. Even when things were going wrong we all believed that my body and my baby's body would always win in the end, even if we needed help along the way.'

One of my least favourite phrases in the maternity dictionary is 'high risk'. You might find that, because of your age, your BMI, an IVF conception or something that happened in a previous pregnancy, a label saying 'high risk' in big, red letters is sneakily stuck to your back or tattooed on your forehead.

Sometimes the 'high risk' label gets applied because of something that comes up in your pregnancy – a possible developmental issue with your baby, extra amniotic fluid or your blood pressure. If your baby decides to show up before 37 weeks, if you are having twins or you've had a previous caesarean, you might find the words 'high risk' being bandied around.

I'm not into labels, and neither are many women I've worked with. Instead of being diverted down a standard pathway, we'll talk about ways to find out what specific risks have increased in your situation. Risk is in the eye of the beholder and you need to fully understand your individual situation. How risky is your risk? Is there anything you can do to minimize it? How might you want to alter (or not) your plans for birth? And in the meantime, if you are having a more complicated pregnancy or birth, feel free to remove any labels from yourself. You are still you and you still get to be in charge of your pregnancy and birth.

If your labour goes off plan it's natural to feel disappointed, and easy to get despondent and passive about what happens next. Remember that you are still the boss and it's still possible to have a good birth. Ask your midwife how you can make this new plan as much like your original one as possible. Get your birth partner to remind you that you can still be active, mobile and have pain relief options. Try putting on some upbeat music to re-energize and re-focus. A dance party in the labour room (even if you are only dancing with your arms) or music during your caesarean (see page 195) can cheer up the whole team.

"

Clare: 'Because my baby was measuring big, my community midwife told me that I was "high risk" and shouldn't give birth at home. This sudden spanner in the works was really upsetting.
My last birth had been difficult, my baby had been big and it hadn't gone well and this one was supposed to be bigger. I didn't want to do anything to put myself back in that position or do something reckless, but I also was trying to avoid the kind of care I'd had in hospital last time. I managed to speak to a really experienced midwife in the team. She took some time to understand my situation and the reasons why I wanted to be at home. She talked me through specific risks of having a "big" baby if there are no other complicating factors.
My community midwife was worried about shoulder dystocia – the baby's shoulders getting stuck after the head is born. But it became quite clear to me in this conversation that I wasn't really at greater risk of anything. Having a suspected big baby is only one of the number of circumstances that increases chances of shoulder dystocia, and birthing at home actually decreases the chances of it happening. My baby was likely to be big because I am a tall woman and the kind of birth I was planning was minimizing my chances of the baby getting stuck. The experienced midwife was really supportive of my plans for home birth and so I decided to go ahead. In the end my baby was a bloody enormous 11lb 3oz. He was born at home and I didn't even tear.'

Emergency caesareans

" Priya: 'It was the polar opposite of what I wanted and
planned for. And I think I get to feel sad about that.
But it was also absolutely the right thing. Everyone was
kind, upbeat and it was still very much a joyful birth.
Him coming out of my stomach instead of my vagina
doesn't make me feel any less of a mother. So there!' **"**

If you are considering requesting a caesarean in advance for
non-medical reasons, or if you have been recommended one
in advance because of a particular medical issue, you'll want
to read pages 195–9.

Emergency caesarean sections have a vital role to play in
saving the lives of women and babies. In an emergency situation it is incredible how quickly and efficiently a baby can be
born and how the team spring into action like a well-oiled
machine to get you and your baby to theatre – and out again –
swiftly and safely.

THE BASICS

'Emergency caesarean' is often a bit of a misnomer. Contrary to
its panic-inducing title, the majority of 'emergency' caesareans
(EMCS) happen in non-emergency situations. Any caesarean
that is not planned well in advance is classed as an EMCS, so,
if you are in labour for a couple of days, resting comfortably
with an epidural sited, your baby's vital signs are perfect but
your labour has simply stalled, you may decide it's time for a caesarean. With no great hurry (and it could take a few hours if the
theatres are busy), you'll be taken in to have a straightforward
and relaxed caesarean birth. This will still be called an EMCS.

The reasons for unplanned caesareans vary wildly. One of

the most common is when labour is not progressing in the way that is expected and when interventions to try and get it to do so (such as synthetic hormones, or changes of position) don't do the trick. A caesarean is often recommended if the baby is showing some signs of distress (a low or fast heart rate or thick meconium in the amniotic fluid), or if, during the pushing phase, not much progress is made.

MAKING THE DECISION

If you weren't planning a caesarean, but one is recommended or suggested as an option, it can be difficult to get your head around and can be upsetting. You usually have plenty of time to discuss this, and a sensible first question to ask is to clarify whether this is an emergency situation. In the vast majority of cases it won't be, and then you can feel free to ask for privacy and time to talk this through with your partner.

Use the BRAIN acronym (see page 223) to help you work out what questions you want to ask your team. It's important to ask these questions so that you're making a fully informed decision and, when you reflect on your baby's birth, you know that you made the decision yourself and why. Research shows that this is an important part of feeling good about a birth that didn't go to plan.

If this is a life-threatening situation, knowing that will often help you make a fast decision. You still always have the right to ask for time to consider and to get information from your caregivers and weigh your options up, no matter what the situation.

GETTING READY

If you decide that a caesarean section is the right option, an anaesthetist will come to talk to you. They will take you through a scary-sounding list of the risks of the procedure (though note how rare many of these complications are) and will often ask you to sign a consent form. In order for your consent to be lawful, they also need to make sure you understand any risks and benefits that are important to you, so you should expect to have a two-way conversation and not to simply be asked to sign the form.

You will usually be given some medication to swallow to help settle any stomach acid. If you aren't going straight into theatre you'll also be advised not to eat or drink anything from now on.

If you're not yet wearing a hospital gown you will be given one before you go to theatre. These delightful garments make it easier for the team to do the operation and attach the various monitors to you as well as protecting your own clothes.

Personalizing your caesarean

When you talk through the operation with your team, let them know anything that is important to you. Do you still want to discover the sex of your baby yourself? Would you like it to be quiet at the moment of birth and for your baby to hear your voice first? Are the theatre staff able to play music of your choice? Can your partner bring a camera to take pictures? Feel free to talk to your team about what they can do to make this feel as close to your original birth plan as possible.

Your midwife may want to shave the top of your bikini line if it's likely to get in the way of the incision. You can ask to do this yourself with privacy, or ask your partner to do it if you prefer. Nobody else needs to be in the room while you have your bikini line shaved.

GOING TO THEATRE

Depending on the situation, you might be wheeled on the bed, in a wheelchair or walk yourself to theatre. Your partner probably won't be able to come with you until after the anaesthetist has finished getting you comfortable in theatre (see below). This can be a difficult and stressful time for your partner and they may want to phone a friend for support. Do make sure they put on their theatre scrubs before you have to leave, as this is usually a sight to behold and a laugh can be pretty helpful around now.

IN THEATRE

When you get to theatre, if you don't already have an epidural sited, you will go through the process on page 147 but instead of an epidural you will be given a spinal block. This is a much stronger drug to ensure you don't feel any pain. Your anaesthetist will check you can't feel anything, usually by spraying something cold on your skin. It's important to be honest and, if you can feel the spray, speak up.

The midwife who has been supporting you in your labour will be there in theatre to look after you. You are likely to be on quite a narrow bed at this stage and you'll have an intravenous drip attached through a cannula in the back of your hand. The anaesthetist will also want to place a (painless) clip on your finger to monitor your vital signs. You can ask for this to be put on your toe instead, so that your hands are less encumbered if you want to hold your baby later on.

Your partner will join you before the operation starts and will sit next to your head. Ask them to help you stay calm and distracted. There will be lots of other people in the room and the team could include:

- Your midwife, to look after you and do basic checks on your baby once it is born.
- A consultant obstetrician or registrar, who does the surgery.
- The obstetrician's assistant.
- A paediatrician, if you are under general anaesthetic, or if your baby will need special care once it's born.
- A paediatric resuscitation team, in case your baby needs help straight away.
- An anaesthetist, who gives you the drugs to numb you.
- An anaesthetic nurse or operating department assistant.
- A scrub nurse, to help the obstetrician with the instruments.
- One or two theatre nurses.
- Medical students or student midwives, though only with your permission.

If you are having twins, or if your baby is expected to need lots of help at birth, there could be more people in the room, but expect 9 or 10 people to be there for a straightforward caesarean.

THE BIRTH

Your doctor will start by making an incision of between 10 and 20cm long around the top of your bikini line. It won't be long until your baby is born. In emergency situations your baby can be out in 2 minutes, though it will take around 10 minutes if there's less of a hurry. Lots of women find the sensations of pulling, tugging and rummaging odd and unsettling, but it shouldn't feel painful.

You might find that the strong spinal block drugs make you shake quite violently. This is normal, but pretty weird. You may find it helpful to use the breathing practices (pages 35, 159 and 274), tension release exercise (page 46), or whatever breathing or coping mechanisms you've been using in labour to help distract and calm you.

Drapes will be put up to screen you and your partner from any view of the operation. You can ask for the drapes to be dropped if you wish to see your baby being born and they will then be put back up.

Traditionally babies born by caesarean section have their cord clamped and cut immediately and are taken to a small, equipped trolley called a resuscitaire to be examined, dried and wrapped up in towels before being handed to the parents – usually to the partner.

There is increasing awareness that skin-to-skin contact is beneficial to both mother and baby. So, if your baby doesn't need any help breathing, and you want to do skin-to-skin, your midwife should help you tuck your baby inside your gown to keep it warm. See Charlotte's story on page 195 for inspiration.

Sometimes your reaction to the spinal drugs, or your need to concentrate on keeping calm, can mean that you don't feel up to holding your baby yet. This is absolutely fine, and if this happens to you then your partner can hold your baby close to you so you can see it and stroke its face if you like.

The rest of the operation can take 30 to 40 minutes.

RECOVERY

Once the caesarean is finished you'll be wheeled into a dedicated recovery area until you are stable enough to be transferred to the postnatal ward. You'll probably feel a bit out of it and strange, though you shouldn't feel much pain at this stage.

If you haven't fed your baby yet, the recovery room can be a good place to do this, or (depending on how long you are in recovery) you can wait until the postnatal ward if you and your baby aren't ready.

After a caesarean you'll be given some glamorous support stockings to wear for 6 weeks to reduce your risk of deep vein thrombosis. You'll have a catheter in place until your spinal block has worn off and your scar will be covered by a protective covering.

Pain relief

In theatre you'll often be offered a morphine injection, a suppository or a diclofenac suppository to provide pain relief for several hours – all of which are compatible with breastfeeding.

You should have a range of pain medication options open to you after birth, regardless of whether or not you are breastfeeding, and should be encouraged to ensure you are taking enough painkillers so that you can begin to move around to feed and look after your baby. If you are breastfeeding, then opiate drugs like morphine are still available to you, but, as they can make some babies excessively sleepy, keep an eye on your baby after feeding. If it is reluctant to feed or wake, then considering another painkiller might help.

> **"** Alice: 'After my first caesarean I thought I'd be all brave and limit what I took. My midwife was really encouraging me to have more than ibuprofen but I thought I'd tough it out. Bad idea. The pain suddenly hit me like a truck in the middle of the night – presumably when the spinal and the "I just had a baby" high had worn off. It was quite difficult to get it back under control. Second time around I just made sure I kept on top of it and then cut down gradually as suggested. It was so much more manageable that way.' **"**

Crash caesarean

In a real emergency you might need a 'category one' or 'crash' caesarean. You can expect things to happen very quickly, and your partner should help ensure that you know what's going on and have time to ask questions, though this time is likely to be limited. During a crash caesarean the team are trying to get the baby out as quickly as possible, so will often offer you a general anaesthetic rather than a spinal block. This means that you will be unconscious when your baby is born and will meet it when you wake up in recovery.

Your partner and birth partner won't be allowed to come into theatre with you if you have a general anaesthetic, but they should be swiftly informed when the baby has been born so that they aren't worrying. If the baby is doing well it will often be brought to your partner to hold while your operation finishes.

It can be really difficult to come to terms with missing the moment of birth, and a crash caesarean can be traumatic for you and your partner. Your partner and team can help by:

- Taking photos in theatre for you.
- Taking photos of the baby meeting your partner.
- Not passing your baby around to friends and relatives before you have held it.
- Delaying weighing, dressing and measuring your baby until you are awake and alert.
- Putting your baby on you, skin-to-skin, as soon as possible.
- Talking to you when you have woken up to ensure you understand what has happened and why. Ask to see your doctor if they don't come to see you.

Assisted birth

Ventouse is a suction cup placed on the top of the baby's head and is only used when you've pushed the baby down far enough. As you push during contractions the doctor will use the suction cup to pull and ease the baby out. There are different sized and shaped cups. The smallest, often called a 'kiwi cup', can be a handy tool to give you a little help as the baby emerges. You often won't need to go to theatre and this can be done in your labour room. Ventouse is usually chosen when the baby is quite far down and the obstetrician is confident that only a little help is needed to help it out.

Forceps are two metal instruments, shaped a little like salad servers. They are lubricated and then inserted into your vagina around your baby's head. There are different sizes and types of forceps and the procedure is usually done in theatre, though in an emergency situation or if you have a preference for staying where you are, you might stay in the labour room. Forceps may be suggested if your baby is a little higher and more strength is needed. Your doctor might offer the option of trying forceps before a caesarean section if your baby is low enough.

For first-time mothers an episiotomy, or cut to the perineum, will almost certainly be needed if you are having an assisted birth, and many second-time women will need one too.

If you are having an assisted birth you should be given adequate pain relief. Gas and air may help, particularly if you are having the smallest ventouse cup, but if you do not have an epidural sited then you should be offered one. You should also be given a local anaesthetic before an episiotomy. If there is a pressing emergency situation you still have the right to wait for an epidural but may want to consider the quicker option of a pudendal block. This is a local anaesthetic injected at strategic points around your vagina and perineum so that it gives fast pain relief to these parts of your body.

> During an assisted birth, ask your partner to stand next to your head and relay any instructions and information from the midwives and doctors to you, and help you stay calm.

Alternatives

As with all interventions, you can decline an assisted birth, no matter what the circumstances. If neither you nor your baby is in distress, you may wish to discuss other alternatives to get the birth moving.

Alternatives could include:

- More time – it might not be 'failure to progress' but 'failure to wait'.
- Different positions – even if your mobility is limited by having an epidural on board. See pages 137–43 for suggestions.
- Thinking about how to get the atmosphere right to help your contractions get stronger (see page 164).
- Asking for help with pushing. Finding it hard, not sure what to do? Talk to your midwife about the different ways she could coach you.

Breech

Your baby changes position lots in pregnancy, but towards the end of the third trimester most babies will helpfully settle into a head-down position with their back towards your front. About 3 in 100 babies will remain bottom or feet down by the time they are considered full-term.

Turning your breech baby

If your baby is breech at 36 weeks you'll be offered an external cephalic version (ECV) to manually turn it. The success of this can depend on the position of your baby, but is also shown to be very much linked to the experience of the practitioner. It's worth finding out what the success rate of your obstetrician is and trying to get booked in with the best pair of hands in the hospital. You'll be offered medication to relax your uterus, which has been shown to make ECVs more successful. On average 1 in 2 babies is successfully turned by an ECV, and there is a small risk of the procedure distressing your baby and/or leading to you going into labour or needing an EMCS.

If you want to try and turn your own breech baby, there isn't a whole lot of evidence to support any particular method. However, some women swear by moxibustion (related to acupuncture), carefully adopting a knee-to-chest or upside-down position regularly to encourage your baby to turn, or undergoing hypnosis.

If you decide not to have an ECV, or it doesn't work, you should be able to choose between having a caesarean section or a vaginal birth. It was previously thought that caesarean sections were the safest way for breech babies to be born, but there is an increasing change in that thinking, and some of the evidence that caesarean recommendations were based on has been discredited. Unfortunately many areas are now seriously lacking in midwives and doctors experienced in facilitating a vaginal breech birth in a 'hands off' way. The 'hands off' approach (which allows a vaginal breech birth that's progressing well to happen without any intervention) is thought by many to be the safest way for vaginal breech babies to be born.

If you want to explore your options you'll find some breech birth resources on www.rebeccaschiller.co.uk/noguilt. If you want to have a vaginal breech birth, your hospital should support you. If they don't have midwives experienced and confident in vaginal breech birth you may want to consider a unit where they do, or ask your local clinical commissioning group or Trust to bring in a specialist midwife to train their staff and/or support your birth.

Back-to-back and other positions

The ideal position for a baby to be in during labour (making it easiest for the baby to move through your pelvis) is head down, chin tucked and back against your stomach. Babies can be and are born in a variety of different positions. One of the most common is back-to-back, where the baby's back is against your back rather than your front.

Being in a less ideal position can make some labours longer and more difficult. Back-to-back labour (also called occiput posterior or OP labour) can cause backache and make it harder for your baby to tuck its chin in and rotate through your pelvis. Remember, though, that most babies who are back-to-back at the start of labour are turned by the contractions, and I've been at a few very straightforward back-to-back births. Try to alternate remaining active with getting some rest. Use all four positions on page 143 for your comfort, and be aware that the early part of a back-to-back labour can be the hardest.

Transverse

If your baby is transverse – lying across your uterus parallel to the floor – it can't be born vaginally unless it turns. You might be offered an ECV, and if your baby is still transverse after that, or you decline it, you'll be offered a caesarean before you go into labour.

Positioning

Upright, all fours and open pelvis positions can help get your baby into a good position. Consider swapping a chair for a birth ball in the third trimester and going for regular walks.

There are lots of resources for discovering more about getting your baby into the ideal position, exercises you can try (before and during labour), and lots of theories about the minutiae of foetal positioning. If these make you feel more confident, do check them out: www.spinningbabies.com is a good place to start. It's also worth remembering that things that switch on the anxious and over-analysing parts of our brain don't tend to help labour. So if you think you might become a bit fixated on perfect positioning, it might not be something for you to explore in depth.

Group B Streptococcus

Two in 10 women in the UK have Group B Streptococcus (GBS) bacterium in their vagina and/or bowel. GBS carriers don't know or feel any ill-effects from these bacteria, and most pregnant women with GBS won't know they carry it and won't pass it to their babies. If it does get passed from mother to baby during birth it is most likely to have no effect. Only 1 in 2,000 babies in the UK is diagnosed with a GBS infection after birth and, though most will recover fully with antibiotic treatment, it can be serious. One in 10 infected babies will die, and 1 in 5 could have long-term issues.

Women aren't offered routine testing for GBS in the UK. If your circumstances mean that your baby is more likely to develop an infection (if your waters broke more than 18 hours before labour starts, if you go into labour before 37 weeks or if you have a fever in labour), you are likely to be offered antibiotics. You can still often use the birth centre if you are having IV antibiotics (though you may be recommended to use the labour ward) and women with IVs have had water births. A senior midwife should be your first point of call (both in advance of labour or if you decide to have antibiotics during labour) if you want to discuss labour options if you are having antibiotics. And if you want to be tested for GBS there are private tests available; see www.rebeccaschiller.co.uk/noguilt.

Meconium

If you notice green, brown or black in your broken waters or on your maternity pad it might be a sign of meconium. Your midwife will offer you monitoring to see whether your baby is coping with labour and will also look at the fluid to see if it is very thick or just a little stain. If you have thick meconium and your baby is showing signs of distress, your team will talk you through revised options for your birth. Remember, if you are well past your due date, meconium could just be a normal sign of your baby being more than ready to be born, so use the BRAIN tool on page 223 to help make decisions about any change of plan due to meconium. In some rare cases babies can breathe (or 'aspirate') meconium into their lungs during the birth. This can cause serious complications, so your baby will be monitored more closely after birth if meconium has been spotted.

Induction

Induction of labour (when labour is started artificially) is one of the most common interventions in childbirth in the UK. Nearly a quarter of women have an induction, often because they go past their estimated due date. You might also be offered an induction for a range of other reasons, including: being over 40 years old, being pregnant as a result of IVF or fertility treatment, concerns about the size of your baby (too big or too small), gestational diabetes, or waters breaking and labour not starting within 24 hours.

In this section I'll look at the standard pathway an induction can take. Do remember that practices vary from hospital to hospital, and you should expect and ensure that your midwife explains exactly what will be offered to you if you decide to be induced.

Mairead: 'I felt positive. Thanks to the induction, contractions were happening. I found some stairs to walk up and down and got labour going a bit more. Four hours later and I'd dilated a bit and was ready and happy to have the drip. I tried to manage without the epidural, as I really wanted to be mobile, but I realized quite quickly I needed it as there was a sudden jump in pain.

The anaesthetist did a mobile epidural that worked really well. I could still stand if I leant on someone, sit on the ball and move around with a bit of help. Very quickly I was fully dilated and I could feel I needed to push.

The pushing was such hard work. It took nearly 2
hours but, as I was making steady progress, I didn't
feel hassled to change plans. The midwife suggested
different positions and I ended up on the birth stool.
I was purple in the face with sweat streaming down
me. My husband was encouraging me and I was just
roaring and going for it. Eventually I felt her head
with my hands and it gave me the last bit of strength
to push her out. Holding her, after all that, was an
insane feeling. Crazy and amazing.'

THE BASICS

As the NICE guidelines make clear, induction of labour can
be an important tool in getting you and your baby to the end
of your pregnancy safely, but it comes with some risk. Women
generally report less satisfaction in their births, find them
more painful, and often feel less in control and more frightened. Caesarean section rates are very slightly lower than in
spontaneous labours, but the rate of assisted births is higher.

When you are offered an induction for any reason you'll
want to get good information from your team to ensure that
these risks are balanced by the benefit to you and your baby
of your pregnancy ending as soon as possible.

**HOW AN INDUCTION FOR BEING OVERDUE
(OR 'POST-DATES') WORKS**

- You'll be offered at least one membrane sweep if
  you go past your due date. If you go for it, your
  midwife or doctor will insert their fingers into your
  cervix, attempting to sweep their fingers around
  the membranes releasing prostaglandins which help

to soften and ripen the cervix and bring on labour. There's evidence that a sweep can increase your chances of going into labour. For some women it feels like a reasonably low-key intervention that can help tip them over into labour and avoid a proper induction. Others find sweeps uncomfortable or painful, and some women find it triggers a tiring period of cramping and spotting but no labour. If you want to decline a sweep you absolutely can.

- Inductions are often offered between 9 and 12 days after your estimated due date, depending on the protocol at your local hospital. Your midwife/ doctor should explain that most women will go into labour by themselves by 42 weeks, why this induction is being offered, any particular risks and benefits for you, exactly how the induction will be performed and give you the chance to ask questions. You can decline induction and NICE best practice guidelines and instruct midwives and doctors to respect your decision. Remember the BRAIN decision-making tool on page 223.
- If you decide to go ahead with an induction you will be asked to come into the hospital, usually first thing in the morning, with your bags and your notes. If the hospital is busy there may be a wait to get started, and if it looks like your induction is not going to happen on the day you come in, you might want to discuss going home for a good night's sleep in your own bed rather than waiting overnight on the antenatal ward and getting tired before things have even begun.
- The induction will usually begin with a period of monitoring to check that all is well with you and

your baby. You will be offered a vaginal
examination and in most cases a drug, usually
delivered via a pessary (a bit like a tampon), is
inserted into your vagina. Some work over a period
of 6 hours, others over 24 hours. With some
pessaries you may be able to go home overnight, so
ask about your local options. The pessary should
start getting to work softening and opening your
cervix and may even start labour. If your cervix is
already open, you might skip this step and have
your waters broken instead.

- This is still labour, so remember all the tips, tricks
and tools to get your environment right, maximize
your calm triggers and minimize your stress
triggers. Mobilizing can help lots too – remember
those stairs we talked about? It's time to find them!
- After a defined period you'll be offered another
vaginal examination. If your cervix needs a bit
more time you may be eligible for another pessary.
If it has already opened, but you have not gone into
labour, your midwife will suggest breaking the
waters. For some women the pessary is enough to
get into active labour. If this is you, you may well be
able to use the birth centre and/or birth pool if that
is part of your plan.
- If you decide to have your waters broken this will
be done with a small hook, inserted through your
cervix to nick the amniotic sac and break it. You
might feel like you've wet yourself and contractions
may well get a lot more intense. You can continue to
help the progress of your labour in exactly the same

way as if this was a labour that had started all by itself. Don't get into the patient mentality – your body and mind still have a vital role to play in this labour.

- After a period of around 2 hours after your waters have broken, if you aren't yet in established labour you may well be offered a hormone drip to bring on stronger, longer and more regular contractions. And after discussing the risks and benefits in your particular situation with your team, you can agree, decline or delay.

- If you decide to have the drip now or later, synthetic oxytocin will be given to you after a cannula is put into the back of your hand. Some midwives will recommend that you have an epidural sited at the same time, as synthetic hormones can bring on sudden and strong contractions. This is entirely up to you and some women do manage without.

- The drip will be started at a lower dose and turned up gradually until labour is strong and established. You will need to be continuously monitored, as babies can become distressed by the sudden intensity of labour. If this happens, the drip will be turned down again.

- Your labour will then carry on through the first and second stage, just like a labour that has started all by itself. Read Chapters 9 and 10 to remind yourself of how your body and mind can work together to help your baby be born.

- The same basic process is followed for other inductions too.

ALTERNATIVES TO INDUCTION

1. **Expectant management** is what best practice guidelines say you should be offered if you decline induction. This includes regular monitoring of you and your baby until you go into labour. If the monitoring picks up any complications, you should be offered a new conversation with your team to discuss this new situation and make a decision about what to do next.

2. **Acupuncture:** There's not enough evidence to say that acupuncture definitely helps bring labour on, but there are some promising signs in some small studies. Some NHS hospitals offer acupuncture clinics for pregnant women. If yours doesn't, you can find therapists who are really experienced in inducing labour.

3. **Sex:** If you feel like having sex (and your waters haven't broken), then, who knows, it could tip you into labour. Prostaglandins, found in semen, are also used in induction pessaries, though you'd have to have a lot of sex to match their levels. Orgasm, and the related release of oxytocin, can often set off contractions. Feeling happy and relaxed, as we all know by now, is good for labour and will hopefully cheer you up!

4. **Eating dates:** Forget pineapples and spicy curries. A small 2011 study showed that women who ate 6 dates per day for the 4 weeks before their

due dates greatly reduced their chances of needing an induction.

Checklist

1. Are you 'high risk'? Make sure you understand why, and get your midwife to talk you through the particular risks and benefits of different birth options in your situation so that you can make good decisions about if, when and how to change your birth plan.
2. Read about emergency caesareans (see page 232), no matter what kind of birth you are planning.
3. Do you know what an assisted birth is and what the alternatives might be? (See page 240.)
4. If an induction (see page 247) is being offered, make sure you understand why, and what any alternatives (page 252) might be, to help you make your decision about what's right for you.

Part 3

Afterwards

Chapter 15

Timeline of the first week

First hour

Meet and greet

Most babies are now placed directly on their mother's abdomen or chest. So if you want or need something different, let your team know. Your baby already knows your voice and the sound of your heartbeat. It will now spend some time learning about your face and smell.

Third stage

Clamping and cutting the umbilical cord and birthing your placenta usually (but not always) happens in this first hour. All your options are laid out on pages 216–20.

Checks and balances

Most routine checks can wait until the end of this first hour, so you can enjoy this 'golden hour' (see page 284) with your newborn.

First feed | A baby left to its own devices takes on average 54 minutes to latch on and start breastfeeding. There's no rush! If you are bottle feeding from birth, follow the same feeding cues to know when to give the first bottle. See page 296 for feeding information.

First day

Vitamin K | You'll be offered a vitamin K injection during your baby's first 24 hours. More information on vitamin K here: www.nct.org.uk/parenting/vitamin-k.

Nappy | Your baby will probably only have 2 or 3 wet nappies and one meconium dirty nappy during its first 24 hours.

Meconium | Your baby's first poos are thick, black and tar-like. Expect one to two poos in the first day. Wipes are useless on meconium – try cotton wool and water or washable wipes.

Clothes · When your baby is against your bare skin (see page 284) it only needs a nappy and a blanket or towel over both of you (heads out!). Make sure the blanket isn't between your bodies. If you want to put your baby down in its crib you'll need to dress it. Aim for as many layers as you are wearing plus one. Hats aren't recommended indoors.

Feeding · During the first 24 hours your baby is likely to want to feed every 1 to 3 hours (see page 312).

Sleeping · The first 24 hours is often a sleepy time. After the initial getting-to-know-you session, many babies put in a good sleep. This is your chance to catch up on rest – take it!

Pain management · If you are in pain from a tear, episiotomy or caesarean you should be offered proper pain relief. See page 286 for more information.

First week

Feeding · Your baby's feeding pattern may change a lot in this first week. See page 291 to get a heads-up on what to expect. Don't forget to make time to eat real, nutritious food yourself.

Sleeping · There will likely be less of this than you would like, and you'll be learning your way of coping and developing strategies (see page 277).

Going home

If you've given birth in hospital you'll likely be coming home with your new baby during this first week. Expect to be offered a speedy discharge in under 24 hours if everything has been straightforward. Remember that they won't let you leave without a car seat.

Midwife visits

Depending on when you go home and how you are doing, a midwife will come and visit you at least once in your first week – much more if you have a home birth or are discharged quickly. If you need more support, don't be afraid to ask for it.

Milk coming in

Whether or not you choose to breastfeed, your milk will come in, replacing colostrum around the fourth day after birth. Expect to feel all kinds of odd and emotional and have mega boobs this day (see page 279).

First trip out

You can take your baby out and about as early as you like or wait for weeks. Start with a small and close-to-home trip and listen to your body if it tells you to go back to bed.

Visitors

Depending on the visitor, guests can be cheery bringers of food and love or a royal pain in the perineum. Set some ground rules in advance.

First poo (you, not the baby)
Post-birth (caesarean or vaginal) the first poo can feel like a big deal. Keep eating fibre and don't put it off too long. Use your breathing practice, relax your jaw, place a box under your feet for optimal poo positioning and give yourself lots of time.

Pain management
If you are in pain, speak to your midwife and ensure it is well controlled. Sudden cramping, clotting, stomach pain or smelly discharge could be a sign of infection, so do get checked out immediately.

Chapter 16

Your Body

> ❝ 'One day I sat in a restaurant when a woman passed by my table with her infant carrier in tow. As she lifted it up to fit between the tables, her shirt raised and I saw that, although she was at a healthy weight and her body was fit, she had that same extra skin hanging around her belly that I do. It occurred to me that a post-pregnancy body is one of this society's greatest secrets; all we see of the female body is that which is airbrushed and perfect, and if we look any different, we hide it from the light of day in fear of being seen. What if the next generation grows up knowing how normal our bodies are? How truly awesome would that be?' – Bonnie Ratcliff, who runs the Shape of a Mother project. ❞

You are not an elastic band. Over the past 9 months your body has – mind-blowingly – grown a human inside it. Your organs have shifted upwards, your blood supply has increased, your hormone levels have altered wildly. Your joints have relaxed, your muscles have separated and you have laid down more fat. You hair, skin, nails, skin pigmentation and gums have changed.

Even though your belly no longer contains a baby, your

uterus is still enlarged, your skin has stretched around it and it may, very reasonably, bear the marks of this speedy expansion. Your body has been through the most phenomenal set of changes. You cannot and should not feel the need to 'snap back'.

Over the course of our lives our bodies change in response to what is happening to us, where and how we spend our time, the food we eat, the exercise we do. In the summer I freckle. In the winter I develop an oh-so-attractive blue-tinged pallor. At times I have been strong and had muscles. At others I've been plumper, softer and less likely to succeed in that sprint for the bus. My body and yours have changed in response to the lives we've been living, but at no other point have they changed as much, and as quickly, as right now.

To a greater or lesser degree the story of your life is written on your body. Any outside pressure to erase the pregnancy part of that as quickly as possible is nonsense. It's part of you.

Raising a body positive kid: Danni, from the Chachi Power Project

'It's never too early to start raising a body positive kid – especially as it encourages you to be kind to your new body. Introduce your babe to people of all genders and colours and abilities and shapes and hairstyles. Help them recognize the person behind the body. Remind them that all bodies are a part of nature and nature is beautiful, therefore all bodies are beautiful. And that also means no more being negative about your own body in front of them. You are their idol, they will mimic everything you do, especially the negative stuff, so NO MORE!'

Realistic expectations

❝ Emma: 'I was totally shocked that the bump didn't go down straight away. I couldn't fit into any of the stylish loungewear I had purchased for the lovely time I was going to have swanning around postpartum. Which also didn't happen.' **❞**

Expect to look pregnant, albeit decreasingly so, for a while after birth. If you are reading this before your baby is born, make sure you've factored an expanded waistline, and a pair of much larger breasts, into your postnatal wardrobe. I'd strongly encourage you not to put any pressure on yourself to return to your pre-pregnancy clothes for a while. Expect to continue in your maternity wear for at least the first couple of months.

It will take up to 8 weeks for your uterus to shrink down to its pre-pregnancy size, though it will take your skin considerably longer. You are likely to have a 'linea nigra', or dark line, going down the middle of your belly for up to a year after birth. Eight out of 10 of us get stretch marks during pregnancy, but these should start to get less noticeable towards the end of your baby's first year.

On www.rebeccaschiller.co.uk/noguilt you'll find links to body positive websites, books and social media accounts. Check these out to see what postnatal bodies really look like and begin to understand how normal and brilliant yours is.

Bleeding

**❝ Alice: 'For the first few days I always sat on a towel or
one of those incontinence pads I'd bought for my
home birth bag so that I didn't get blood on the sofa.
I did have a few leaks, so I'd suggest dark, loose, old
trousers and pants at first. I used proper maternity
pads at first and switched to ordinary sanitary towels
within the first week. The flow was pretty light by
the end of the second week and I stopped bleeding
entirely by the third week – apart from a bit of
spotting if I went for a long walk.' ❞**

No matter how you gave birth, you will start to bleed quite heavily afterwards. Your midwife will keep an eye on you to ensure your bleeding isn't over the top. If you've been lying down for a while you can expect a sudden gush and/or some small clots when you stand up, but you shouldn't be soaking a maternity pad in under an hour. If you are, tell your midwife pronto.

This discharge (called lochia) is like the mother of all periods, as your uterus empties after 9 months of work. For the first couple of days the lochia is mostly made up of blood, but increasingly it is biased to other tissue from the lining of the uterus. As time goes on, as well as getting gradually lighter in flow, your lochia gets lighter in colour.

> You may well find that if you over-exert yourself in those first weeks your bleeding becomes heavier in response. Consider this a sign from your uterus that you need to slow down.

Hormones

" Sophie: 'I was blown away by what the birth
hormones did to my brain. I was the newborn:
everything looked and felt different.' **"**

Your hormones have been working overtime in pregnancy
and they haven't stopped yet. While you are busy dialling
down on the pregnancy hormones, the internal chemistry
connected to breastfeeding and motherhood is now kicking
in. New mothers experience massive hormonal changes post
birth, and understanding them can help you make sense of
why your body might behave differently for a while.

Your oestrogen and progesterone levels, which have been
raging away in pregnancy, now take a nose dive. Prolactin
levels also drop slightly, but as the drop in progesterone is
much more significant (and progesterone stops prolactin
from doing its thing), it can now get to work. As well as
having a big role in milk production (pro + lactin = pro lactation), prolactin encourages your body to keep storing fat
and lowers your sex drive. Thanks to the joys of prolactin
you might also find that your vagina is less lubricated post-
natally and while breastfeeding. Prolactin can also interfere
with dopamine (which is important for making you
feel happy) and can make you feel less energetic.

Your oxytocin levels will have been particularly high
immediately after birth, and you'll retain higher than usual
levels of this hormone for a while whether or not you are
breastfeeding.

Given all that's going on, you will feel the impact of the veritable hormone conference happening inside you. Effects include: mood swings, feeling irritable, sudden fits of crying or joy (especially around when your milk comes in), skin breakouts, loss of interest in sex, hot or cold sweats (particularly at night), retaining fat stores while breastfeeding, falling to sleep more easily after breastfeeding, losing the extra hair you've grown in pregnancy.

New fathers also experience hormone changes in pregnancy and after birth. If your partner is a man, his testosterone level will have come down and his oestrogen, oxytocin and prolactin levels will have increased. There don't seem to have been any studies on female partners but I'd be willing to bet that your girlfriend or wife won't get through the postnatal period without experiencing some hormone shifts too.

Breasts

Whatever your feeding plans, your breasts will have changed significantly during pregnancy. The map of veins under your skin will have become more visible, your breasts will have got larger and may have started leaking colostrum. Your areolae (the circles around your nipples) will have darkened dramatically and enlarged, becoming targets to enable your baby (whose vision is largely based on black and white at first) to find your nipples and latch on after birth.

Weight

I remember standing on the scales a few days after my daughter was born, excitedly anticipating being nearly back to my pre-baby weight. Ha ha! All of us lose the chunk of weight related to our baby, placenta and amniotic fluid at the moment of birth. But don't be surprised if the scales don't tip to the left that much. Women quite often retain a lot of water in the week after birth. This is often most noticeable if you've had IV fluids in labour or had a caesarean section, but I swelled until my eyes looked like two tired raisins pressed into dough after a straightforward vaginal birth. Top tip: don't let your partner choose the super swollen day to take a charming 'mother and baby' photo to be circulated to all your colleagues. Mine is still paying off this debt.

Breastfeeding, tiredness, prolactin levels and disturbed sleep patterns all impact on our eating habits and metabolic rate. Your body has deliberately stored fat for breastfeeding, and if you switch yourself into a calorie deficit too fast you will be left at risk of burnout, fatigue, and it can impact negatively on your mental wellbeing.

> If you are breastfeeding you can eat as normal – there are no foods to avoid – but try to make sure you are eating enough protein and calcium. The latter is particularly important, as otherwise breastfeeding might deplete your calcium stores and up your risk of osteoporosis later in life. So eat more dairy or alternatives such as fortified milks and fish with bones.

Remember that being sleep-deprived impacts on your appetite and what you want to eat. Research confirms what my postnatal biscuit habit made me suspect: being tired makes it harder to make 'healthier' decisions. Your brain will crave high-energy options – simple sugars and fats.

If you've recovered from an eating disorder or have a current eating disorder, you may want to get some support or clinical help as you adjust to your postnatal body and cope with the challenges it may bring.

Exercise

If you've had a straightforward birth, be led by how you feel – there's no specific time to avoid exercise or goal to aim for. Gentle walking and yoga – when you feel ready – can help you feel less tired, but if your bleeding increases in response to whatever you are doing, take it as a sign you need to kick back. I confess that my entire postnatal exercise regime consisted of walking to the coffee pot and an increasingly desperate swaying motion to persuade my daughter to sleep.

If you've had a caesarean you'll want to wait until you've seen your doctor around 6 weeks. More serious tears and stitches will also need you to wait a while before doing anything higher impact.

Sex

" Fran: 'The main issue was milk shooting out of my boobs like water pistols whenever I was turned on. Took some getting used to!'

Lisa: 'I did not feel like having sex for a long time. I was busy, tired, emotional and sore. It took 6 months to persuade myself to try it and she was a toddler before I felt like we'd found our groove again.'

Emma: 'Pregnancy and birth have changed my body sexually for the better. I enjoy penetrative sex much more than I did, and my nipples (which were sensitive and responsive before) have become much more so.' 🙸

It's normal not to feel like sex for a while after birth – especially if you've had a tear or an episiotomy. There's some evidence that waiting at least 3 weeks for vaginal sex is a good idea, but if you have a tear or stitches you'll want to wait until they are healed, as sex is an infection risk. There's of course no reason why you can't get busy with non-penetrative sex in the meantime, though you might not feel super sexy right now. Don't feel under pressure to return to sex until you feel up to it. The *British Journal of Obstetrics and Gynaecology* reports that only 4 in 10 women had vaginal sex by 6 weeks post birth, and 2 in 10 hadn't got back in the saddle by 12 weeks (see www.rebeccaschiller.co.uk/noguilt).

Checklist

1. Check out what postnatal bodies really look like so you can be realistic about your expectations (see page 264).
2. Give yourself a break about your postnatal weight, and read about why it might not be a good idea to

focus too much on shifting the pregnancy pounds
(see page 268).

3. Work out what postnatal exercise feels right to you
and how you'll get help to fit it into your new life
(see page 269).

Chapter 17

Your Mind

After I'd had my first baby I was high as a kite for about 3 weeks. Shattered, yes, my brain working slowly, forgetting words and putting porridge oats in the coffee pot. But the overarching emotion was hysterical joy, mixed with light fear and lurking knowledge that we'd got ourselves into something bigger than we could have imagined. It was when my husband returned to work that I found things harder. But I was lucky and had good support, coming back up to the surface quickly after any lows. There's a chance you'll feel exactly the same but, more likely, you will have your own very different journey through the glistening peaks and dark valleys of these days and weeks.

Your emotional wellbeing after birth is dependent on a raft of interrelated factors: how the birth went, whether you are in pain, how much sleep you are getting, whether you had antenatal depression or a pre-existing mental health condition, how confident you are feeling about feeding and how well you feel it's going, the people you have around you and – as we discovered in Chapter 16 – your reaction to the crazy hormonal party happening inside you.

For Annalise, the early days of new motherhood were full of love:

" 'I was absolutely ecstatic, probably for weeks. I had so much energy that I couldn't rest for a while. I couldn't stop looking at my baby and I felt so much love for my partner. I was also really proud of myself. Most things went to plan and those that didn't we dealt with together. I found it much more difficult having a toddler than a newborn!' **"**

For Anne, after a difficult birth, things were darker.

" 'If I let myself talk about feeling sad I was afraid I'd really lose it, and I felt a responsibility to keep it together because I was a mother to a baby now who needed me. I didn't feel like I could talk about it at all. It was the weirdest thing. I wouldn't let my family visit. I felt that I couldn't share their happiness and I didn't want to ruin it for them, so if I couldn't put a brave face on it, I shouldn't see them at all.' **"**

For many women feelings are more complicated. There's absolutely love, joy, wonder and pride, but often mixed with anxiety, confusion, tiredness and a bit of panic. You can expect to feel all the feelings that you've ever felt, all at once and more intensely than ever, just like Millie did.

" 'I was thrilled with the baby and doing that new mum thing where I thought he was the most beautiful baby in the world by far. I was recovering well, really happy in so many ways, but then I'd get waves of terror about him not getting enough to eat or being too hot. I was beyond tired and just kept bursting into tears all the time. I'd find myself staring into space in the middle of a task having no idea what I was doing.'

Breathing practice 3: Alternate nostril breathing

This is particularly good for sleeping issues and can feel rejuvenating.

1. Close your eyes if that feels OK. Breathe normally in through your nose and out through your mouth.
2. After a couple of breath cycles, gently place your index and middle fingers of one hand in between your eyebrows.
3. Use your thumb or ring finger (depending on which hand you are using) to close off your right nostril. Inhale through the left nostril.
4. Then use your thumb or ring finger to close your left nostril and exhale through the right nostril.
5. Inhale through the right nostril. Then close that right nostril and exhale through the left. Inhale through the left then close that nostril and exhale through the right.
6. Continue for 5 to 10 breath cycles.
7. Before you open your eyes and finish, do 3 normal breaths.

Why you might feel a bit weird

Hormones: If you think PMT makes you act a little odd, wait until you've experienced the far greater surges and drops in hormones that happen after birth.

Lack of sleep: If you've lost sleep during your baby's birth, then this, added to the interruptions in sleep a newborn is guaranteed to bring, can make you feel below par. Short temper and a difficulty focusing are really common. The less sleep you have the more fogged your brain will be; it can be hard to concentrate and even simple decisions can be overwhelming. Tiredness can make you feel low and can impact on your immune system, making you more susceptible to germs. Finding ways to sleep can make a big difference. See page 277 for tips.

Pain: If you are in pain this can have an impact on your mental wellbeing. You are more likely to be tense, breathe in a less relaxed way and your body's reaction to pain may cause chemical responses, making you feel stressed. Insist that your midwife helps you get your pain under control.

The shock and awe of the new: You may not have held a baby before and now you are charged with looking after one. Even if you've already had a baby, this is your first experience with this many children and with this baby. Many women talk about the overwhelming shock and awe at this new, all-encompassing experience. Some women experience feelings of regret that they have chosen to take this path. For Ellie, who had been trying for four years to have a baby, the regret was a huge surprise:

" 'I'd been desperate for a baby for so long and was completely certain I would only feel happiness. I was happy and relieved but I was also terrified. It didn't feel the way I was expecting it to. I remember thinking that I'd made a terrible mistake and actually saying to my girlfriend that I was regretting the whole thing. I actually felt better once I'd said it – guilty but better. And 3 years later I know that it was just a wobble.' **"**

What helps

The basics: It can be easy to forget to eat, drink, go to the toilet, wash and sleep in the early days. You still need to do these things to feel human and keep yourself in basic shape for the days ahead. Set yourself an alarm, or ask your partner to remind you, to eat 3 meals and some snacks every day. Go to the toilet every couple of hours, particularly if your bladder is feeling numb from the birth. And prioritize having a shower or bath – every day if you can.

Support: You need a team – especially if you don't have a partner. Consider hiring a postnatal doula who will boost your confidence, have lots of tips, listen to your hopes and worries and do some basic cooking and tidying. If you can afford it, or if family can pay for one as a gift, get a cleaner for the early weeks. If you have family and friends who have offered to help, tell them what you need and, if they are reliable and won't drive you mad, take them up on their offers. Ask them to: cook food for you and drop it round, pop round to help with housework, washing and ironing. If visitors want to hold your baby (and you are happy for them to), use this hands-free time to wash, nap, eat or get 10 minutes of fresh air rather than make small talk. Tell your partner what you need them to do in advance, and remind them if they forget. If you've traditionally done most of the household chores, this balance needs to change, at least for a while, though ideally for ever. Speak to your midwife, your health visitor, your breastfeeding counsellor, as appropriate. If you don't have anyone to turn to in person, online forums such as Netmums, Mumsnet and local parenting forums can be a source of virtual support. There are a number of helplines for feeding, mental health and other kinds of support on www.rebeccaschiller.co.uk/noguilt.

Resisting google: Online forums are one thing, but frantic, obsessive googling of your infant's every move does no one any good. Seek support from real people and from the books and forums you trust.

Exercise: Getting back to some light exercise can help counteract some of the physiological stuff that might make you feel tired, sluggish and low.

Talking: Feeling low? Tell someone – now! Your partner, your best friend, your midwife, your GP. If you aren't ready to tell someone in person, take a look at www.rebeccaschiller.co.uk/noguilt for lots of online and telephone support. Remember that 8 in 10 women feel low in the first couple of weeks after birth.

Sleeping: Getting enough sleep is the holy grail of new parenting. There are lots of different strategies and, as time goes on, you'll discover what works for you. In the first weeks after birth your baby will wake often in the night to feed. Expect to feel very tired, and plan how you will manage without an uninterrupted night's sleep. Try sleeping in shifts by going to bed early after the evening cluster feeds (see page 302) and getting a 2 to 3 hour head-start on shut-eye while your partner or supporter looks after the baby. Try napping in the daytime too. The breathing practices on pages 35, 159 and 274 can help you feel sleepy during daylight hours.

Sleeping safely

To minimize the risk of Sudden Infant Death Syndrome, make sure to read the SIDS Prevention advice (www.nhs.uk/conditions/pregnancy-and-baby/pages/reducing-risk-cot-death.aspx). The safest place for your baby to sleep for the first 6 months is in the same room as you.

Research also shows that most parents fall asleep with their babies at some time or another. It can be hard not to when you are very tired and your baby settles better close to you. Falling asleep accidentally with your baby on the sofa or chair is very dangerous. Studies suggest that if you are formula feeding, are a smoker, have a high BMI, have a premature birth or have taken drugs or alcohol, then it also isn't safe for you to sleep with your baby in your bed.

But if you don't tick those boxes and follow some simple rules about bedding, planning to sleep with your baby in your bed regularly, or on nights where they won't settle in their crib, might help you establish breastfeeding more easily, get more shut-eye in between feeds, and prevent you accidentally falling asleep with them on the sofa. Read more about safe sleeping and co-sleeping at the Infant Sleep Information Source, www.isisonline.org.uk.

Day 4 (or 2 to 5)

Day 4, or somewhere thereabouts, is the classic time for a hormone crash. It also coincides with the time when your adrenaline and any post-birth euphoria is wearing off and the effects of a few sleepless nights have kicked in. To top that all off, whether you are breastfeeding or not, your milk is coming and your breasts will feel full and sometimes hard and sore. For many women this day is really tricky. You may feel happy one minute, anxious, crying or sad for no apparent reason the next. You may suddenly doubt your ability to be a mother, argue with your partner, be cross with your older children or lack confidence in your feeding.

This is all normal and it should pass reasonably quickly. When you, your partner and those around you know in advance that day 4 can be a difficult day (and that it may well happen on day 2 or day 5!) they can be ready to be understanding and help you get through the day.

Helping yourself

Whatever your previous experience of mental wellbeing, prioritizing looking after yourself in these first weeks as a new mother, especially the hidden, emotional aspects of yourself, is vitally important. It's easy not to – after all, looking after what goes on inside our head is not something we have been told to prioritize.

I hope that you have already started to get into positive habits and become committed to making yourself a priority.

This all needs a bit more thought and dedication now that you have added looking after your new baby into the mix.

It is inevitable that you will have less time to focus on your needs as you get used to new motherhood, but the work you've done in pregnancy will have helped enormously.

Every day: Find a window of time for yourself. Ideally 20 minutes, but 5 minutes can work too. Do the breathing practices or the tension release exercise (page 46) if you only have 5 minutes. Try a yoga practice if you have longer. Or one of the mindfulness apps on www.rebeccaschiller. co.uk/noguilt might be more your cup of tea.

If you are feeling overwhelmed: Try the breathing practices, the tension release exercise or the anxiety mindfulness exercise on page 282. Tell someone. Consider making an appointment with your GP, or talking to your midwife or your health visitor.

Every week: Do one thing that you love that has nothing to do with having a baby. Suggestions: meet a friend, read a bit of a book, have a bath with bubbles and candles, watch a TV series you've been meaning to watch for ages, masturbate, buy some new lipstick/clothes, have a haircut, do some exercise, make a cake, start a journal, read a bit of a magazine, plan your new business/next career move/novel.

Tell your partner how important it is for you to have some space and time, even 5-minute windows, to check in with yourself. If you are doing this on your own, get support from others to have this time to yourself, or take the chance when your baby is sleeping.

Postnatal mental illness

Baby blues: Baby blues isn't a mental illness, but simply another way to refer to the really common feeling of being low, anxious or overwhelmed after your baby is born that happens to most women. This should start to lift and you should feel gradually more like your old self within a couple of weeks. It's very normal to have low moments throughout parenthood (heck, throughout life), but if you feel persistently low or it is getting worse, read on.

Postnatal depression (PND): It's pretty common to have PND, and 1 in 10 women experience it in the first year of their baby's life – some even find it starts when their babies are toddlers. That rises to 4 in 10 if you are under 20 years old. It can creep up on you gradually, so keep an eye on how you are feeling and make sure your partner is aware of the signs of PND so they can encourage you to seek help if you need it. These include:

1. Feeling sad or low a lot or all of the time.
2. Lack of enjoyment and loss of interest in the wider world.
3. Feeling tired all the time and not having any energy.
4. Having trouble sleeping at night.
5. Difficulty bonding with your baby.
6. Not wanting to see friends or family.
7. Finding it hard to concentrate or make decisions.
8. Intrusive thoughts, which are often repetitive, for example, about hurting your baby by dropping it.

Anxiety: We can all feel anxious as new parents, but if you find yourself experiencing panic attacks, feeling a persistent sense of worry, being constantly concerned about your baby and dwelling on the negatives, you might be suffering with postnatal anxiety and it's time to seek help from your GP.

> **Mindfulness**
>
> While you wait for an appointment it can help to practise some mindfulness when your mind gets overtaken with anxiety. Concentrate on the detail of something you can see: the wallpaper, a piece of fabric, a pattern in a wooden floor. Focus your entire mind on the item you are looking at. Take in the tiniest of details. Slow your breathing gradually while you focus on it.

Intrusive thoughts: We all have intrusive and unwanted thoughts at some time in our lives. Have you ever been at the top of a tall building and had a sudden flash of throwing yourself off or falling off? On my first walk with my newborn daughter, pushing her pram beside a canal, I was plagued by thoughts of tripping and her falling in. It's common to have occasional intrusive thoughts in life and in early parenting. But if these thoughts become relentless, repeated or distressing, they could be a sign of PND, OCD or another postnatal mental illness. If they are bothering you, seek help.

PTSD: If you have had a distressing or traumatic experience during childbirth, you might experience fragmented flashbacks, nightmares and feelings of sadness, anger or fear. Trauma symptoms and post-traumatic stress disorder can be brought on by a traumatic birth or another trauma in your life. If you are struggling with symptoms such as these, please see your GP and www.rebeccaschiller.co.uk/noguilt.

Postpartum psychosis: This very rare condition affects only 1 in 1,000 women after birth. It is more common in women who have a history of mental illness, particularly if they have experienced psychosis or bipolar disorder. Symptoms start in the days after birth and can include hallucinations, mania, psychotic episodes and delusions. Immediate psychiatric help is urgently needed, but the condition is very treatable and, with help, the outcome is good. Most women will need to spend time as an in-patient and many are able to attend a mother and baby psychiatric unit so that they aren't separated from their babies.

Checklist

1. Make time for a breathing practice after your baby is born – every day if you can (see page 274).
2. Be prepared for the 'day 4' hormone crash, and make sure your partner is too.
3. Talk about your approach to sleeping with your partner and read the SIDS and co-sleeping safety guidelines (see page 278).
4. Commit to carving out time for yourself every week and get your partner on board (see page 279).
5. Know what postnatal depression symptoms to look out for (see page 281).

Chapter 18

Your First Week

The first hour

> **Susannah: 'I scooped her up from the birthing pool and cradled her in my arms and felt an epic, life-changing, all-consuming, world-redefining love – more intense than I ever could have imagined. Still brings tears to my eyes thinking about it.'**

In the first hour after your baby is born, time can move in the slow-yet-lightning-fast way that accompanies the most important moments in our lives. If you and your baby are doing well, you can expect to spend this hour getting to know each other.

This time of connection is often called the 'golden hour'. As doula and breastfeeding counsellor Maddie McMahon explains: 'After birth, both the baby and the mother need to rest, safe and warm in skin-to-skin contact with each other. The mother's oxytocin levels are off the scale; this hormone of love contracts her womb, helping her birth her placenta and preventing her bleeding too much. Over the first hours, oxytocin floods her brain, causing her to fall in love with her baby – and the baby, lying calm and cosy on her chest, is awash with the love hormone too, bonding them with their mother, regulating their temperature, heart rate and respiration.'

What will happen immediately after birth?

You or your midwife will probably bring your baby straight on to your chest unless you request otherwise or the baby needs some help with breathing. In the UK, babies are no longer routinely washed after birth, and as little wiping as possible should be done so that the protective substance called vernix, which coats your baby's skin, stays put.

Your midwife will keep an eye on your bleeding and general wellbeing, as well as watching to see that your baby is gaining a good colour and breathing well.

You are likely to need to give birth to your placenta (see

page 216) during this first hour. You can hang on to your baby while you do this, or pass it to your partner.

If you are bleeding significantly from a tear in your perineum, your midwife will suggest examining this and stitching you. If you aren't having heavy bleeding you may want to wait until that first hour is over to be examined, as some women find this painful.

Your baby will eventually be weighed and measured by your midwife and offered a vitamin K injection at some point soon after birth. A paediatrician (or midwife or GP if you have a home birth) will do a full top-to-toe check on your baby in the first few days.

Tearing and stitches

Unless you have a caesarean you will be offered an examination after birth to check for tears. If you don't have an epidural on board this can be really sore, and your midwife should offer you gas and air if you would like it. She will look and feel around your vagina, anus and perineum to see if you need any stitches. I had a lovely gas-and-air-fuelled daydream about my new baby while my midwife checked my perineum and I didn't feel a thing!

Between 6 and 7 out of every 10 women who give birth will need some stitches – though the majority have less serious tearing that can be quickly repaired using a local anaesthetic. Being stitched shouldn't hurt, and if it does, feel free to shout for more local anaesthetic.

If you have a small tear that isn't bleeding much it may not need stitching at all, so if you'd prefer not to be stitched, ask your midwife if this option might work for you.

If you have a third or fourth degree tear (one that extends

into your anus), you will be offered a spinal anaesthetic and the tear will be repaired in theatre by doctors. You'll be offered a course of antibiotics and some laxatives.

> ### Recovering from a serious tear
>
> It can be difficult to be open about any long-term problems (such as pain, painful sex or continence issues) following a tear. Though these problems are relatively rare, women who have them often find it difficult to get support or are too embarrassed to talk about it. You can have treatment so it's important to speak up. Tell your midwife if you are still under her care or your GP if not. If your problems persist you should be referred to a gynaecologist and/or a specialist physiotherapist. There are resources to help on www.rebeccaschiller.co.uk/noguilt and the Women's Postnatal Health Community Facebook group can provide good support.

If you tear at a home birth, midwives will stitch you at home – using the same local anaesthetic as in hospital – unless you have a more serious tear, which will need a transfer to hospital.

If you had an episiotomy this will also need stitching. Episiotomies can be more painful and take longer to heal than tears. But whether you simply have swelling or grazing from birth, a tear or an episiotomy, you can expect to feel very tender for at least the first day or two after birth. Between 2 and 4 in every 10 women find their tear painful for up to 12 days after birth, but fewer than 1 in 10 will report longer-term pain.

What if your baby or you need some help after birth?

If your baby is born needing some help breathing, this can sometimes be done with the baby on your chest, allowing it to benefit from the oxygenated blood still flowing into it from the placenta and ensuring that your first moments after birth are still as a united unit.

Otherwise, the cord will be clamped and cut and the baby will be taken to a specially equipped trolley called a resuscitaire, usually in the same room as you, where it can be given oxygen, its vital signs can be monitored, and its breathing will be stimulated. If your baby is expected to need assistance, the paediatrician will usually be called into the room before the baby is born. Unless this is a sudden emergency situation, you will usually have time to discuss this in advance with the doctor, let them know what's important to you and ask what's feasible in terms of getting the baby into your arms sooner rather than later.

> It can be scary if your baby is out of your sight. So ask your midwife or your partner to narrate what's happening to you.

If your baby needs to go to neonatal intensive care, or the special care baby unit, ask if you are able to hold it first or (if it is too unwell) whether you can see it before it goes. There are tips for coping with a separation on page 327.

The first day

Amy: 'I just stared at her all day. I don't really remember sleeping, or moving or eating – though apparently I did. I just wanted to drink her in.

**And ring my mum and tell her every last detail
of what she smelled, looked and sounded
like. I was drunk on the baby!'** **"**

The first day with your new baby is likely to go past in somewhat of a blur. Presuming that you and your baby are well and are together, there should not be much for you to do other than get to know each other.

If you are at home or in a birth centre, you will be able to spend some time as a family getting to know one another, and any older children and close relatives should be able to come and visit if you want them to. Visiting restrictions and transferring to a postnatal ward do create a few more obstacles in hospital, though increasingly some units allow partners to stay overnight. Do think about how you'll feel about being separated from your partner when you choose where to give birth, and investigate which hospitals local to you ensure partners can stay overnight.

After an initial period of being awake, alert and feeding (more on feeding on page 296), many babies often have a period of 6 to 8 hours of being very sleepy and recovering from the birth. It's tempting to spend this time awake, gazing lovingly at them, but try to get some shut-eye if you can.

Solo parenting

" *Sophie: 'When someone offers to help, reply
HOW ABOUT THURSDAY? Always take them up on it
and always give them specific times that would work.
Or it won't happen. Your ten kind offers of help will
waft away into dust.'* **"**

Gemma has been a single parent with both her children. She had her first when she was 21. Here are her tips for those of you doing this without a partner:

> **"** *'Make sure you have a stress release. Mine was a call to my mum. I'd phone her and say, "Sorry mum but . . ." then scream, sometimes even cry.'*
>
> *'When you are feeling stressed, take 5 minutes out. Put the baby down in their cot, let them cry if needs be and regroup.'*
>
> *'Every time they achieve a first or do something awesome and they look for you . . . just you! That's the magic. You know everything they have become is down to you.'* **"**

The first week

In the first week of your brand-new baby's life you can expect it to change in personality, looks and behaviour more than once. This is so exciting, but can also feel as if, just as you got a grip on its pattern and needs, it changes into an altogether different creature and you need to start again.

Your baby is developing rapidly and you are fine-tuning your instincts. With the right support and information you will be able to cope and get to know how to respond to this new person. You will have doubts, worries, and every new parent is convinced that they've broken their baby at some point in the first week. Trust yourself – you've got this.

Going home

For most women this first week contains an exciting and nerve-racking journey from birth centre or hospital to home. If you've had your baby in a birth centre or have had a straightforward birth without an epidural, you'll be offered the chance to leave within 6 to 12 hours of birth. If you are keen to get back home and are feeling well, you'll probably be keen to take up this offer. But if you'd like the support of midwives around you, feel free to ask to stay a little longer.

An epidural means you'll probably need to stay in for a little longer as it wears off, your catheter comes out and you get back on your feet. If you've had a more complicated birth or caesarean section, expect to stay in hospital for at least 2 to 3 days.

After the relative sleepiness of the first day, your newborn is likely to 'wake up' at some point on day 2. You may find that it wants to feed more often, and at some point towards the end of the second or third day this can feel almost constant. Know that this is a normal pattern, connected to your milk coming in around day 4 (see page 279). There's nothing wrong with your baby, you aren't doing a bad job – this is what new babies do.

Top tip: A stretchy wrap sling can be a lifesaver if you (like many of us) have a baby who doesn't want to be put down. It can transform pacing round the house, or being trapped under a sleeping baby, into hands-free, cup-of-tea, go-for-a-walk readiness. Many babies find the foetal position, wrapped-up-tight-against-your-heart cosiness comforting, and a quick walk round the block (or your flat) usually sends them straight off to sleep. You can breastfeed in the sling too, once you know how.

My husband used to take our youngest to the pub at 6 p.m. in our stretchy wrap. I'd bath and read to my oldest and then get into the bath myself. He would have a walk (during which the baby would fall asleep), a pint (during which the baby would stay asleep), and then – once the baby woke – he'd walk back. I'd feel refreshed (well, a bit refreshed) and ready for the night. Learn how to tie a stretchy wrap on www.rebeccaschiller.co.uk/noguilt.

Visits and tests

You will see a midwife at home after you are discharged, and they will check that your uterus is contracting, that your bleeding is within normal range, that your baby is feeding well and that you and the baby are feeling OK. You'll be able to ask questions and discuss any concerns and, in your sleep-deprived state, you may find it useful to keep a notepad with questions on the go, as you are bound to forget something when the midwife arrives. You'll be given emergency contacts to call if you are worried about yourself or your baby.

On day 5 after birth you'll be offered a heel prick test for your baby. A small needle is used to prick its heel and drops of blood are collected on a card. These are tested for: sickle cell disease, cystic fibrosis, congenital hypothyroidism and a number of metabolic diseases. You'll get confirmation of a negative result when they are between 6 and 8 weeks old, but should hear sooner if your baby tests positive for anything.

Tips for coping with the first week

- Stock up on freezer food in advance, and accept gifts of food from friends and family.

- Make time to eat, drink and go to the toilet. Resist the temptation to eat only biscuits and choose a high-fibre diet. However you give birth, the first postpartum poo can feel scary, and keeping your bowels moving and avoiding constipation is important.

- Set realistic goals: do not expect to get dressed, do housework, host visitors, cook from a recipe, do any work. Consider staying in bed or on the sofa as much as possible.

- Write a list of queries for when your midwife visits.

- If and when you feel overwhelmed, return to the breathing exercises earlier in the book (see pages 35, 159 and 274).

Checklist

1. Make a 'golden hour' plan if that's important to you (see page 284).
2. Consider perineal massage during your pregnancy (see www.rebeccaschiller.co.uk/noguilt) to reduce your risk of tearing (see page 286).
3. Make sure there's something nice to eat and drink when you get home from hospital. Or treat yourselves to a takeaway, as you are unlikely to feel like cooking.
4. Remember to do your breathing practice (see pages 35, 159 and 274).

Chapter 19

Your Decisions

> Hannah: 'I looked at my incredible son and thought, "Oh shit, I don't want to screw this up." But I took some comfort from the fact that we'd had a pretty rocky pregnancy, with lots of things we had to research and decide on. We'd done pretty well with that stuff so there was no reason we couldn't keep doing a good job for him now he was on the outside.'

Pregnancy and birth are good training grounds for the lifelong series of decisions you can and will be able to make about your child's wellbeing, your lives as a family and how that fits with your needs as an individual. These start the moment after birth.

Placenta

Your placenta is just that – yours. Feel free to look at it, keep it, bury it, eat it, make it into tablets or make placenta prints. Don't give a monkey's about it? That's fine too. For some the placenta holds no interest – having just given birth to a brand-new person, you might be keen to get rid and move on as soon as possible.

If you are interested, there are lots of options for what to do with your placenta after birth. There isn't a high-quality evidence base to support eating or encapsulating your placenta, which may be because there aren't any benefits, or may be a symptom of it not being very well studied. Anecdotally, women who do something with their placenta feel positive about the experience and the effects it has. There are resources for researching your placenta on www.rebecca schiller.co.uk/noguilt.

Feeding your baby

When, what, where and how to feed your baby can feel like a minefield of complicated and emotionally laden decisions to make. This section is here to help. I'm going to encourage you to set your own goals, give you factual information, troubleshooting ideas and tips, and signpost you to expert sources of support. I've also asked women to share their own, very different feeding experiences. I hope you'll see that there is a whole host of choices you can make, that plans can and do change, and that what you actually do is entirely up to you. No one else gets to have a say or is allowed to judge you because of the way you feed your baby. And the most important thing is that you have knowledgeable and caring support around you as you make these decisions.

I've enlisted the help of two experts: Vanessa Christie and Shel Banks. Both have the highest qualification in infant feeding (International Board Certified Lactation Consultants, IBCLCs) and they work with new mothers making these decisions and dealing with the realities of feeding newborns every day.

Do read both the breastfeeding and the formula feeding sections below, whatever your feeding plans. This will help you work out what's right for you, allow you to support friends making different choices and will keep you informed should your goals change.

Breastfeeding

" Rebekah: 'It was surprisingly emotional. I wanted to do it and it was hard and it was all super intense – like I couldn't see the wood for the trees. Thank god for an amazing breastfeeding counsellor at the local drop-in who scooped me up and sorted it out. She told me I didn't have to do this but if I wanted to she would help. Giving me permission to stop helped me carry on. It was actually just a few tweaks to the way I was holding her, learning how to feed lying down (godsend – do this immediately!), that made it all better. And just knowing that I could stop if I wanted to meant we carried on happily until about 10 months.' "

Getting informed

Information is empowering. If you decide that you want to breastfeed, remembering how and why you made that decision can really help to see you through any tougher times. I've put together a basic guide below but it is not comprehensive, so you'll want to look at breastfeeding positions and think about ones that might work for you if you are having a caesarean, are having more than one baby or have movement limitations. Here are some popular positions:

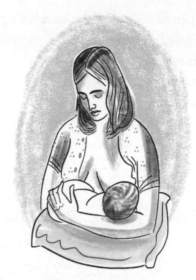

Cradle hold

Feeding lying down

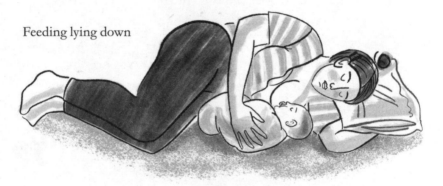

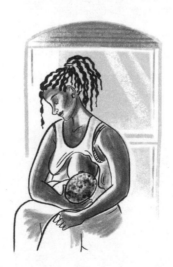

Cross-cradle hold

1. Try different positions to work out what's comfortable for you. Cradle hold, feeding lying down and cross-cradle hold are some ones to try. More laid-back positions might work better for you and your baby. Find out more at www.biologicalnurturing.com.

2. Look at pictures and videos of latching and sucking so you know what to look for. This is a good start: www.nhs.uk/start4life/breastfeeding-videos.

3. Find out about your local reputable breastfeeding clinics, peer support groups, discover what services are available via your hospital or community midwife, and get the number of a local International Board Certified Lactation Consultant (IBCLC).

4. Have a breastfeeding troubleshooting resource. There are some basics in this book, but a dedicated book or website can help with daily queries or questions, as can a support helpline.

5. Set yourself a basic feeding goal for the first 2 weeks and review it regularly. Keep your goal realistic, tailored to your circumstances, support network, other family needs and desires. Examples of 2-week feeding goals include: 'I want to give my baby colostrum and establish breastfeeding effectively so that I can breastfeed exclusively if I decide to.' 'I don't know how I'm going to feel about breastfeeding but I'm going to try it for 2 weeks with no pressure.'

 Ju: 'I found it really tricky to get comfortable feeding her after my section. The latch wasn't good and it was just adding to me feeling in pain. I stopped

after a week. I do still feel guilty about it – the curse of motherhood! I would give it another go next time, but I know it was also the right thing at that time.'

How milk-making works

- During pregnancy the breasts start to make colostrum – a thick, yellow, concentrated source of immune factors, protein and minerals.
- Colostrum is usually all a baby will need in the first few days. It is released in tiny amounts, but is potent and a perfect dose for your baby's tiny stomach.
- After the baby and placenta are born, progesterone levels drop and the process of producing more copious amounts of milk (led by prolactin) starts. This leads to an increase in your milk supply from around days 2 to 5, when the milk 'comes in'.
- Once your baby starts suckling at your breast, nerve endings are stimulated, causing oxytocin to be released and contracting tiny muscles in the breast which push the milk forwards and out of the nipples. This is known as the 'let-down' reflex, and causes some women to feel a tingling sensation, increased thirst or even some pain in the breasts and/or in the uterus. Others may feel nothing at all and only notice it is happening through the change in the baby's suckling pattern – slower, deeper, with pauses to swallow.
- The more often a baby drinks from the breast (and/or milk is expressed), the more the brain gets signals to keep producing more for the future. If the breasts get poor stimulation (if your baby/pump aren't used often or aren't working well), milk production will decrease.

- Breasts are never empty and milk is continually being made as long as the stimulation is there. You don't need to wait between feeds for your breasts to 'fill up'. This has the opposite effect – your body thinks it needs to make less milk. The more drained a breast is, the faster the rate at which it fills up again and the greater the concentration of higher-calorie and fat-rich milk. This explains why women can make enough milk for twins or more.

- If breastfeeding has been going well (or if a mother has been frequently expressing with an effective pump), then a full milk supply tends to be established between 2 to 4 weeks. From this point until the baby is around 6 months, the amount of milk it drinks is about the same, but the components of your breast milk will change according to the baby's needs.

- As long as the breasts are being stimulated frequently (at least 8 to 12 times in 24 hours) and effectively (your baby is actually removing milk), the vast majority of women can produce enough milk for their babies.

- Ensure that, overall, your breasts are stimulated about equally. There's no set amount of time you should feed for (some babies feed faster than others) and some babies take both breasts at each feed, others just one, while some like to do different things on different days. It's normal for your baby to prefer one breast to the other.

- Some women may need extra support and intervention to establish a partial or full milk supply – details on page 310.

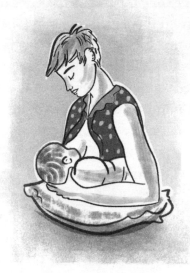

Cluster feeding

It's normal for new babies to have an intense period of short, close-together feeds in the early evening. These are often called cluster feeds and can also happen if your baby is unwell, has had a very long nap or is having a growth spurt. You'll soon see a pattern to these intense feeds and can make sure you have food, water and entertainment to sustain you while they last. The time your baby decides to cluster feed (somewhere between 5 p.m. and 10 p.m.) can feel really gruelling and shocking at first – especially if you aren't expecting it.

> **"** Alice: 'I was expecting it to be all kinds of difficult but we just hit the ground running. She latched quickly and after a few ouchy feeds we got the latch right and that was it. I introduced formula around 5 months to get ready for going back to work and we stopped completely around 7 months. I'll definitely do it again with this next baby.' **"**

Pain

Breastfeeding often feels tender at first, but it should never be grit-your-teeth-toe-curling pain. If you find yourself digging your nails into the bed, always ask for help. Most commonly, pain issues can be solved with changing how you position yourself and your baby. It's most commonly caused by a shallow latch (baby only taking the nipple into the front of its mouth, where it will be compressed, rather than the back, where it won't). Other causes can be tongue tie, thrush, Raynaud's syndrome or a poorly fitting breast pump. If you are told that 'it looks fine' and it still feels awful, ask somebody else.

> **"** Julia: 'I was completely unprepared for how painful feeding would be when my milk came in. After fairly happily feeding for 3 days, I literally felt my breasts inflate and suddenly they were rock hard and I just couldn't latch my daughter on. I didn't feed her for the best part of 12 hours, which is pretty horrifying in retrospect. Eventually I just had to grit my teeth and somehow we managed. The second time around I was prepared for it and just rode out the 10 seconds or so of pain – but I really wish someone had told me what to expect when my milk came in.' **"**

303

Sharing the load

Remember that breastfeeding itself is the only thing that partners and other family and friends can't do to support a breastfeeding mother. However, they can take on any other roles, such as winding, settling, nappy-changing, bathing, dressing and taking the baby for walks, as well as being a general help around the home.

" Rhea: 'My girlfriend basically did everything apart from breastfeeding for the first 3 weeks till she went back to work. My job was to recover and feed the baby – which felt like more than enough. It was harder with our second as I needed to spend time with the older one too, but we kept to the rule as much as possible and it really helped me get on my feet.' "

Vanessa's top tips for breastfeeding

Let's face it, breastfeeding isn't always easy at the start and you should never doubt yourself if it isn't coming naturally. Back in the distant past, when we all lived in close proximity to extended family and helped raise each other's children, we would see someone breastfeeding all the time. Today we live in a very different world, and often feel as if we are somehow supposed to know what to do and feel racked with insecurity if we don't.

Many women and babies take to it like ducks to water but for others it can be a rockier ride, and being focused on the bigger picture in the early days can sometimes feel overwhelming. In these times, it can help to see each day of breastfeeding (and even each individual feed) as an achievement in its own right, and never be afraid to seek out the support you may need to overcome any hurdles that are in your way.

> " Anna: 'I breastfed both my babies. The first time it wasn't smooth sailing after a NICU stay. We used quite a bit of formula until she weaned around 10 months. I was more relaxed and confident the second time and my daughter was born in great shape. Despite planning to mixed feed again, I never got round to it. I'm still happily breastfeeding her at 18 months.' "

1. **Know what a hungry baby looks like**

    A baby opening its mouth, sticking its tongue out, rooting (turning head to side and opening its mouth) and sucking on its fists is telling you it is hungry way before any crying starts. It's usually easier to latch a baby on before it gets to the red-faced wailing stage.

2. **Know that your body works**

    The worry of not having enough milk is a very common reason for stopping breastfeeding. Some conditions can directly impact on a mother's milk production, but the most important factors are to ensure that you are feeding frequently (and/or expressing) and effectively (i.e. your baby is able to remove the milk well from your breasts). These two things guarantee that your brain will get strong messages that the milk is moving and that it needs to put in the orders to make more. If your baby isn't feeding much (and there are plenty of reasons why this might happen), don't hesitate to seek help to get to the root of the issue.

> **"** Julia: 'What kept me going was that a couple of people had said it took 6–8 weeks before they felt really at ease – otherwise I think I'd have felt pretty discouraged at the idea of several more months of what was quite a bumpy ride.' **"**

3. **Know who to ask for help**

Figuring out whose advice to trust can be very frustrating when you are faced with lots of different opinions. Knowing how to weed out the dodgy advice and finding informed, objective and compassionate support is often crucial to success. The best people to speak to in times of need are certified breastfeeding counsellors (who often work for voluntary organizations) or IBCLCs.

4. **Chuck 'guilt' out of the window**

There's something about becoming a mother that immediately allows 'guilt' to creep into practically anything we even dare to think about! We only ever make decisions like these based on what we feel and know to be right for us at the time. If you struggle with breastfeeding and it ends prematurely for you, you may well feel sad (that's normal) but please don't feel guilty. Chances are that you will have done everything within your resources to make it work and you are one hell of an amazing mama.

5. **Wait to express – if you can**

Unless there is an unavoidable reason to express your milk, try holding off for the first month if breastfeeding is going well. This gives your body the best opportunity to figure out how much milk it needs to be making, and also gives your baby a decent amount of time to figure out how to comfortably latch on to your breast and control your milk flow, before possibly introducing any bottles.

6. **If in doubt, go back to basics**

If it all feels too much, go back to basics: skin-to-skin, dim lighting, soothing music, getting in the bath together with your baby (as long as there is another adult around in case you feel weak or dizzy). Know that it's OK not to feel OK when your body is aching, you're exhausted, your hormones are doing hula hoops and you're adjusting to new motherhood. Reach out for support!

7. **Get your partner to help by:**

- Ensuring they are as informed as you are about breastfeeding.

- Checking latch – another pair of eyes and from a different angle can be very helpful.

- Settling the baby afterwards so you can have some time to yourself.

- Getting you drinks and snacks and making sure you always have water and the remote when you sit down to feed.

- Helping you to relax – gentle massage, cuddles and keeping visitors at bay.

- Being positive and supportive and believing that you can do it.

- Much of the above applies just as well if you are formula feeding.

" Mia: 'My baby was born at 30 weeks and couldn't even try to breastfeed for ages as she was unwell and didn't have the instinct yet. I did lots of expressing – at first in the hospital and then rented a hospital grade pump for home. It made me feel better to be doing something and more connected to her. Despite lots of skin-to-skin we never got her to latch and she's always been bottle fed. I do feel sad about it but, in the grand scheme of things, it's been OK. Luckily I'm an expressing demon so she's had breastmilk pretty exclusively until 6 months and plenty more afterwards.' **"**

Where to turn for help if you need it

National Breastfeeding Helpline: 0300 100 0212
Association of Breastfeeding Mothers: www.ABM.me.uk
La Leche League Leader: www.laleche.org.uk or
    0345 120 2918
NCT Helpline: 0300 330 0700

Find a support group near you: www.ABM.me.uk/
    breastfeeding-support-groups
Breastfeeding videos: www.bestbeginnings.org.uk
Find a lactation consultant near you: www.lcgb.org/
Find a tongue tie divider near you: www.tongue-tie.org.uk

Troubleshooting

MILK NOT COMING IN

Some factors can lead to a delay in your milk coming in. These can include how your birth went (IV fluids, emotional stress and exhaustion, large blood loss or incomplete delivery of the placenta) or a history of hormone issues (diabetes, polycystic ovary syndrome, fertility difficulties, hypothyroidism), as well as having a very high BMI.

What to do:

- Be confident that with the right breastfeeding support, most hurdles can be overcome with a variety of different strategies.
- Where possible, seek specialist breastfeeding support from an IBCLC. Some hospitals and community trusts employ IBCLCs and many more work independently.
- Ensure that your breasts are being emptied frequently and efficiently.
- Spend as much time as you want to (and are able to) having skin-to-skin contact with your baby.

- Your midwife and health visitor should keep a close eye on your baby's weight gain and nappy contents. If your baby is not getting enough milk, supplementation with either donor breast milk or formula may be required.

LOW MILK SUPPLY

The most common reason women say they stopped breast-feeding earlier than initially planned is because they felt that they didn't have enough milk. Read the section above on how milk-making works (page 300) to understand the process and what can get in the way.

Some other things can lead to low milk supply. These include:

- A premature birth.
- Hypoplasia, otherwise known as insufficent glandular tissue (IGT) or underdeveloped breasts.
- A history of breast or upper back surgery or injury, including breast augmentation or reduction.
- Some medications (including some hormonal contraceptives).
- Flat or inverted nipple shape.
- Breastfeeding management issues (restricting feeds or poor advice on positioning).

What to do:

- If your baby is losing or not gaining weight (note: it is normal to lose some weight after birth and regain it by around 2 weeks), and not having enough wet and dirty nappies, this could be a sign of it not getting enough milk. If you are worried about your supply, ask to speak to your hospital's infant feeding coordinator, go to a breastfeeding drop-in group, call a breastfeeding hotline or – if problems persist – get assessed by an IBCLC at home. They will assess what's going on, why it's happening and how you can turn things around for the better with strategies such as deeper latching, breast compressions, switch nursing, expressing and galactagogues (herbs and medications that can increase milk supply), among others.

How to know if your baby is getting enough to eat

Most babies lose weight initially, and losing up to 10 per cent of their birth weight is considered normal, so looking at the contents of their nappy is the best way to work out if they are getting enough milk.

In the first 48 hours, your baby might only have only 2 or 3 wet nappies. These should then start to become more frequent, with at least 6 wet nappies every 24 hours from day 5 onwards. Add cotton wool inside the nappy if you are unsure whether the baby is weeing. The urine should be pale and not dark brown.

After the initial meconium, poo turns green and then yellow, and your baby should be doing about 3 yellow poos every day. Babies who fill their nappies at this rate are getting enough to eat. If not, get help from your midwife and breastfeeding support as soon as possible.

BABY NOT FEEDING VERY OFTEN IN FIRST FEW DAYS

As a general rule, gaps between feeding should be no longer than 4 hours from the beginning of one feed to the beginning of the next. If your baby is feeding well every 1 to 3 hours and has one gap of 5 hours, it's very unlikely to be an issue. If a new baby isn't 'demanding' anything regularly because it is extra sleepy, wake it every 2 to 3 hours for a feed.

MASTITIS

Mastitis is an inflammation in your breast which might be due to an infection or a plugged milk duct. You'll notice redness and a tender spot or sore lump in your breast. If you feel well in yourself, it is likely to be a plugged duct from milk not draining properly. If the redness spreads, the breast feels hot, pain is intense but localized and you feel unwell, it is likely to be caused by infection.

What to do:

- Warmth (hot water bottle, getting in the shower or bath) and breast massage, then breastfeed the baby and/or express. The key is to keep the milk moving. Stopping feeding will make it worse.
- Rest: go back to bed (with your baby if you know how to co-sleep safely), eat, drink and get some help with older children or household tasks.
- Loosen any tight bras or clothing and have someone who knows their stuff check how the baby is latching and complete a breastfeeding assessment.
- If after 12 to 24 hours of doing this the symptoms are the same or worsening, see your GP, who will most likely prescribe antibiotics.

FEEDING AFTER A CAESAREAN

If you have an epidural/spinal anaesthetic and your baby is well, it is possible to breastfeed immediately after a caesarean – even in theatre. If you need a general anaesthetic, it may take a little longer until you have recovered sufficiently. Always ask for help, as you may need it to get in a comfortable position for feeding. The first few feeds are likely to be with you in a reclined position, and will be made much easier with some extra hands to assist you and your baby. If you know you'll be having a caesarean, ask if your partner or a supporter can stay with you on the postnatal ward to help you outside visiting hours.

What to do:

- Women often find feeding in the 'rugby ball' position helpful, to keep little feet away from the scar. Lying on your side in bed with your baby lying alongside you on the mattress can also be a good post-caesarean position.
- Your baby may be sleepy from the effects of any pain relief or anaesthesia. If it is not showing much interest in suckling in the early days, have someone show you how to hand express (see www.rebeccaschiller.co.uk/noguilt) and feed your baby colostrum via a syringe at least every 2 to 3 hours. You may need to wake the baby up and encourage it to feed. Keep your baby close to you and it will start suckling when ready.
- If you needed IV fluids during labour, this may over-exaggerate your baby's post-birth weight loss, since they will have taken in some of this fluid through the umbilical cord.

- Sometimes (but not always) it can take a little longer (an extra day or two) for your colostrum to turn into more copious amounts of milk. Check that the frequency of wet nappies is increasing, that your baby is having at least 2 to 3 dirty nappies each day, and keep offering the breast and/or expressed milk at least every few hours to ensure the baby is getting enough milk in the meantime.

BABY WANTS TO BE FED 'ALL THE TIME'

Babies are born with tiny tummies (small marble-size at birth), which are only capable of comfortably and safely taking small amounts of milk at a time. Milk is also designed to be easily and quickly digested. Babies work on instinct, and their instinct is to feel warm, safe and fed. Breastfeeding provides all three of these things. You can't feed a breastfed baby too much, but make sure you are getting time to eat, drink, shower. This phase is short-lived but intense.

BABY FEEDING FOR VERY SHORT PERIODS
OR VERY LONG PERIODS

If a baby is consistently suckling at the breast for only a few minutes at each feed, or every feed is lasting an hour or more, it is worth seeking specialist support to check things out.

PRESSURE FROM FAMILY/FRIENDS/HCPS
TO STOP BREASTFEEDING OR TO CONTINUE
WHEN YOU DON'T WANT TO

The decision whether to continue, to reduce or to stop breastfeeding is always in your hands. If you are exhausted, upset or in pain, it is understandable for those who love you to want to 'make things right'. The suggestion is often to introduce bottles, which may or may not have been in your original plan. If this is not what you want, being pressured to do so can have long-lasting effects on your wellbeing. If you want to try and find breastfeeding solutions, despite facing bumps in the road, your friends and family can be invaluable in supporting your choice. And anyone who doesn't needs to be kept at a distance for a while. On the flip side, if you have decided that you no longer want to breastfeed and are happy that you have made a decision that feels right for you, everyone around you should support you.

> **Christina: 'Learn to feed lying down after a section! I was expecting it to be more difficult than after my vaginal birth but, apart from needing to adapt the positions for the first week or so, it was no different.'**

Shel's formula feeding basics

During skin-to-skin time after birth, most babies will begin to show feeding cues, such as sticking their tongue out, opening their mouth and turning their head to the side.

If you are exclusively formula feeding, a bottle can be gently introduced at this stage, remembering that babies need very little milk in the first 24 to 48 hours of life as their tummies are tiny. Your baby might not want to feed again for 6 to 8 hours after this, and in a newborn this is totally natural – being born is exhausting! After the first 12 to 18 hours of life your baby is likely to be more wakeful and want to feed more frequently, but remember that small frequent feeds with plenty of pauses are more biologically normal for the baby.

Different hospitals will have different policies on providing milk for newborns. Some hospitals still provide free formula bottles and teats to families who are not breastfeeding. The milk is bought in by hospitals from the companies in small ready-to-feed bottles which have single-use teats to accompany them. This milk is a pasteurized liquid which can be used at room temperature and kept for an hour after opening. It usually comes in 70ml bottles.

In some areas free formula milk is only provided in cases of clinical need – where breastfeeding is not going well or there is some other reason the baby cannot have breast milk. In these hospitals, families are expected to bring in their own formula milk, in small ready-to-feed bottles with single-use teats. This ready-to-feed milk can be stored in your bag until it's needed and is available in most supermarkets. Check with your hospital on its policy in advance.

> **"** Lynn: 'Why didn't I breastfeed? I basically think it's nobody's business. I didn't want to, it didn't appeal and I knew it wouldn't work with my job. I didn't get pressured in to doing it – thank god – and feel totally happy with my choice. Baby seems pretty happy too!' **"**

How often to feed

Newborn babies take only small amounts in the early days. By 10 days they might take 20 ounces (roughly 570ml) in

24 hours, and by 2 weeks they might be taking roughly 26 ounces (750ml).

After the first day or two, babies need to continue to be fed little and often. Bottle feeding increases the chance of overfeeding, because it's instinctive for the baby to keep sucking and swallowing as long as there's milk flowing. Pausing and removing the teat from the baby's mouth from time to time, and possibly breaking the feed up by placing the baby diagonally up on to the adult's left shoulder to see if there's any trapped gas ready to come up, will allow the baby's appetite to catch up with their stomach.

> **Carly: 'I hadn't got on with breastfeeding the first time and was certain I wanted to formula feed my next one from birth. I was expecting some pressure from the midwives but, having put it really clearly on my birth plan, they were absolutely fine with it.'**

Connecting with your baby

Babies love to watch faces, so they want to see the face of the person feeding them. Eating should be a sociable thing, so I'd encourage new parents to engage with the baby while it's feeding, if it's alert. Depending on whether the baby is being mixed fed (sometimes referred to as 'combination feeding') or purely bottle fed, parents might wish to hold and feed the baby in different positions. Regularly switching which side you hold your baby on, and which hand you feed them with, can help with their development.

If your baby is switching between bottle and breast, or being supplemented (perhaps because of weight loss), but where the aim is to get back to full breastfeeding, consider supporting and feeding the infant in as similar a position as possible to a breastfeeding position. Have the baby held snugly next to the adult's body, head tipped back and mouth wide, with the teat pointed up and back into the roof of the mouth, bottom lip and chin touching bottle and nose very much free of the bottle.

Preparation and storage

Follow the Department of Health Guide to Bottle Feeding (2015), which has 14 illustrated steps. It's really important to follow the guidance on sterilizing, powder storage, temperature of water and storage of made-up milk, as poor hygiene and preparation can lead to sometimes serious illness.

Mixed feeding

There's very little 'prescription' or evidence base on which to make informed choices on mixed feeding – feeding a combination of breast milk and formula. If the intention is to breastfeed alongside bottle feeding, get breastfeeding established before introducing bottles. After that, it's really a case of working out what works for your own baby, and your own situation. If you need someone to talk through your situation with, you might want to approach an IBCLC or breastfeeding counsellor.

If you are bottle feeding your breastmilk, make sure you know how to store it safely (www.laleche.org.uk/storing-your-milk).

❝ Lisa: 'I did feel a bit like having "I've had breast surgery" tattooed on my face in the early days. I was very happy letting the baby twiddle about on my breasts. It felt nice, it comforted him a bit and I loved it when he started looking up at me when feeding. We did much more breastfeeding than I'd planned. But we all knew it wasn't going to get enough calories into him. I got a bit sick of feeling like I had to explain it to well-meaning people. So I stopped explaining and just got on with it. He was very happy and healthy and had a mix of breast and formula – though way more of the latter.' **❞**

Troubleshooting

COW'S MILK ALLERGY (CMA)

Formula milk is made from cow's milk, to which between 2 and 7 babies in every 100 are allergic. Symptoms include eczema, problems digesting milk, explosive smelly nappies, severe wind and/or vomiting and lots of crying. If your paediatrician or GP thinks your baby has CMA, you should be referred to a dietician and can be prescribed special formula milk to which it won't be allergic. Many children grow out of this allergy, so speak to your dietician about how and when to consider re-introducing dairy products.

Which milk to buy

Formula milk is strictly regulated, meaning that the contents are very similar regardless of the brand. Many parents choose what is available in their closest local shop and what is most affordable. Ready-made cartons are more expensive, but they can be very handy for feeding out and about and minimize the chances of making up powdered milk unsafely.

There's no evidence to support the claims that 'hungry baby', 'comfort' or 'good night' formula have any benefits. As they are often more expensive and can cause problems for some babies, many parents choose to avoid them.

> Anne: 'I was pretty devastated that breastfeeding hadn't worked out for a whole host of reasons. I stopped completely in week 5 but Bea had been having lots of formula from week 2. I had to grieve for this thing I had been so sure I would do and had felt so strongly about. I did feel a bit ashamed as most of the women I knew were breastfeeding. No one expected me – hippy, home birth Anne – to whip out a bottle. It was necessary but it was hard. Next time I'll seek more support and I will go much easier on myself.'

Checklist

1. Read about your third stage options so you are ready to work them into your birth plan (see page 344).
2. Find out about local placenta services if this interests you (see page 295).
3. If you plan to breastfeed, work through Vanessa's breastfeeding tips (see page 304), using the information on www.rebeccaschiller.co.uk/noguilt

to get clued up on positioning, attachment, latching and sucking. Get yourself one of the recommended breastfeeding books too.

4. Make sure your partner reads the 'How milk-making works' section (page 300). A supportive partner has been shown to make a dramatic difference in women meeting their breastfeeding goals.

5. If you plan to bottle feed formula or breastmilk, make sure you know how to safely prepare and store your baby's milk (see page 318).

Chapter 20

The Unexpected

Life with a new baby is full of unplanned and un-plannable things. If this is your first baby, however carefully you've read this book, however many babies you have hung out with or held, it will feel like another world. Expecting the unexpected, and being ready to flex in response to it, is a key parenting skill that can take a while to develop.

What was the most unexpected thing about afterwards?

Jacqui: 'That after having a big baby, I felt like I'd been run over by a truck. All my bones felt loose and jangly and I felt I was walking like a string puppet!'

Scheenagh: 'How strong my maternal instinct was! I had no experience of children, had never changed a nappy and disliked sprogs intensely as a youngster. But I knew instinctively how to dress, feed and look after our first baby.'

Jacqui: 'That my bladder would be totally numb for 3 weeks after birth. I had no sensation of needing a wee and had to just go and sit on the loo every few hours just to see if anything would come out.'

Jo: 'That the absolute best smell in the world is new baby smell. Forget Chanel No. 5, Jo Malone candles and all that crap – there is nothing quite like sniffing your baby's head! Oh god, that sounds so weird.'

Rosie: 'That I could actively resent people for having had a full night's sleep. It was like they were smugly radiating this "I've slept well" vibe, and I couldn't believe I'd ever feel like that again.'

Anucyia: 'That I wouldn't be able to poo! Constipation was a real problem and hard to overcome. When I finally did, nearly a week after my daughter was born, it was unflushable and my boyfriend ended up boiling a kettle to "melt" it away.'

Seren: 'How close and loving I'd feel with my partner. They had been through so much with me and we now had this little person shared between us. I was smitten with the family unit, not just the baby!'

Becky: 'Nobody warned me about the afterpains with my second, third and fourth child. They were worse than childbirth.'

Elizabeth: 'It was easier than I expected. I loved almost all of it.'

Jess: 'I remember being shocked at the pain I was in after a vaginal birth. Everyone talks about the joy that comes after childbirth but not the soreness, the pain from stitches, not being able to sit properly, the fear of using the bathroom. I wish someone had told me I'd be very hormonal and in a lot of discomfort.'

Deborah: 'The sense of being so connected to another human being that I wasn't quite sure where she ended and I began. I remember going to the GP leaving her behind with my partner and the image of her face was burning in my mind.'

Fran: 'How different babies can be. First barely slept in his first week and second slept so much that I was convinced he had been starved of oxygen at birth and suffered brain damage. I genuinely asked the health visitor if it was possible.'

Natalie: 'How many vases I had as opposed to how many bouquets of flowers I received! All lovely of course but nowhere to put them after the first three!'

Clara: 'The terror! That I would drop her down the stairs, that she would stop breathing, that no one else was capable of looking after her.'

Sian: 'My second daughter did a funny reflex crawl up my body to find milk just after she was born. I was utterly stunned and amazed by nature. I had thought this was just a story from cloud cuckoo land made up by the antenatal teacher.'

Kay: 'The total shock/realization I felt when I picked up the phone to make a hair appointment, 3 days after coming out of hospital, then putting it down again realizing that I could never just think of myself ever again.'

Julia: 'No one talks about the hot flushes you get at night-time post birth! I was drenched in sweat.'

Kay: 'That not everyone feels that overwhelming love thing. My first thoughts were: concern – is he OK? – relief – thank God he's here – and worry – OMG, how am I going to cope? I just felt an overwhelming sense of responsibility and tiredness and pride.'

Pam: 'How no one in real life actually got judgey about me formula feeding. I kept waiting for some imaginary hippy mafia to jump out on me in the supermarket but they didn't. None of my breastfeeding friends seemed to get any gip for feeding in public either.'

Reena: 'That I'd get really angsty when other people held her.'

Lisa: 'The excitement and generosity of virtual strangers to me. Just general goodwill flooding our way. When my son was born prematurely we'd come home to find a friend had left meals on our doorstep, and she kept going for almost 2 months.'

Catherine: 'My breasts leaking (badly) while I was asleep. I thought I'd burst a hot water bottle in the bed, it was so soaking wet.'

Emma: 'The husband HATRED. I remember kicking him as he slept next to me while I tried to latch the baby on to my bleeding nipples.'

Helen: 'That nappies are supposed to do up at the front!'

Amy: 'The overwhelming love – the ultimate natural high! Honestly, after it wore off I tried to google oxytocin and considered buying it online.'

Caroline: 'That their stomach is the size of a marble when they're born. It helps you not to worry as much about how much (or how little) they eat.'

Sarah: 'That I felt so emotionally raw, like I'd been born again as a new person. Or as if I had been "peeled" of my old personality. Everything made me cry, even how his eyelashes grew every day, or how tiny his nostrils were. I genuinely thought he was the most beautiful baby in the maternity ward, and felt truly sorry for all the other mums whose babies were so boring and ugly.'

Erika: 'When I was pregnant I read all the baby books
I could get my hands on. It came as something of a
shock to realize after a few days that the baby clearly
hadn't read the same books.' **"**

Being separated from your baby

Being parted from your new baby is incredibly hard. Even if
the separation is for 30 seconds, the emotional distress it can
cause can't be underestimated.

Having read this book I hope that you and your birth partner
will be in a good place to ensure that any separation is absolutely
necessary and that, if at all possible, you and your newborn are
kept together after birth. It is always worth asking whether any
treatment that requires the separation of you and your baby can
be achieved in a similar way while keeping you together.

For example, many hospitals routinely treat babies who
have more serious jaundice by placing them under special
lights. While the treatment is usually effective, it can be distressing for a mother who can't hold her new baby. Ask your
hospital if you can try using a biliblanket, which offers light-
therapy via a blanket which wraps around the baby. This way
your jaundiced baby can get the treatment it needs in your or
your partner's arms.

Coping with separation

Doula Maddie McMahon suggests you think oxytocin. Send a T-shirt you've worn with the baby so that your smell goes with them. Your partner's voice will help soothe the baby, so they may want to accompany the baby to the special care unit. And, when your partner returns, make sure they bring photos and videos of the baby. These will help to reassure you and will also help stimulate your body if you are expressing colostrum.

If you are expressing for a longer time, then items that smell of your baby, videos of your baby or expressing at the side of its cot can really help the milk to flow. Just thinking about your baby can help.

What helps most is great support. When families experience challenges on their journey, they sometimes need more than nature can provide, because nature has been interrupted. Skilled, specialist feeding support can be crucial to help them jump the hurdles. Just as importantly, the family need loving care and nurturing, as they may have been through a scary or traumatic time.

Kate's story

(Which talks about the death of one of her sons and her journey to breastfeeding his brother.)

> 'My baby and I were dangerously ill after birth; he was born at 32 weeks and I was in a coma, so I didn't get to meet him until he was 6 days old.
>
> Before that my husband, with the help of one of the nurses in intensive care where I was being looked

after, hand expressed some of my milk on to a handkerchief and put it into the incubator with Henry so he would know the smell of his mother.

I clearly remember the nurses rushing up to us as we arrived in NICU one morning in about week 2 and saying Henry had started making sucking noises. From that point on I was determined to breastfeed. The nurses were very supportive and I did kangaroo care [where a baby is cared for in skin-to-skin contact against their mother instead of in an incubator, often with amazing results] almost all day every day. During this time he was tube fed and he was still very small, so we had to be really patient. It was excruciating.

I was encouraged to express and they would put anything I could give to Henry through the tube. The first few times I expressed, milk had come out but as the days went by it was less and less. I was mourning the loss of Henry's twin brother Thomas (who died at birth), processing what we were learning about Henry's brain damage day after day and my body was trying to recover, so, in hindsight, it is really not surprising that I wasn't producing much milk!

We took Henry home, on the bottle, a week before his due date. I continued to just put him near my breast hoping as he got stronger he might latch. He would latch and suck a little but it was definitely not enough. I was doing it just to feel close to him and I was resigned to this being the way we did things. We noticed he had a tongue tie which we thought might be contributing to things and my doula suggested a lactation consultant. When the consultant came to see us and snipped the tongue tie everything changed. After that visit we were able to stop bottle feeding and exclusively fed him at my breast. Amazingly it worked. He kept steadily gaining weight and he carried on breastfeeding until 14 months.

It definitely helped us bond, it gave us time to get to know each other and I felt like we had worked together to make it happen. I really didn't know that you could start to feed so long after birth. With my two girls (born after Henry and Thomas) there seemed to be so much pressure on me in the first hours to get a good latch and feed – like if we didn't manage it straight away it wouldn't happen. Henry's story shows that isn't always the case.'

Premature birth

If your baby is born before 37 weeks it will be considered premature. You'll be advised to give birth on the labour ward in case the baby needs help with breathing immediately after birth, and will be offered steroid injections to help mature its lungs. Many babies over 34 weeks are born at a good birth weight, and, though your team will keep a really close eye on them, many later pre-term babies don't need very much in the way of additional support and can often remain with you without going to special care.

Sometimes even later pre-term babies need more help, and if your baby is under 34 weeks they are very likely to need some additional medical support after birth. The smallest babies, those under 30 weeks, may need considerable support and will likely spend many weeks or months in hospital before being discharged. If you go into labour before 24 weeks, your team will explain to you that your baby cannot survive outside the womb this early. There is a section of this book dedicated to miscarriage, stillbirth and the death of a baby, and you'll find that on page 331.

Sha's second baby was born at 33 weeks.

" 'It was totally out of the blue – my first had been full-term. I was absolutely bricking it but everyone was really reassuring. The birth was quick and pretty easy. Turns out it's not quite such an effort pushing out a 4 pound baby! I'd got to chat to the paediatrician first and they said she'd be passed straight to me but that if she wasn't picking up they'd cut the cord and take her to the resuscitation table. It was an anxious few minutes but she was basically born pretty fighting fit. She stayed with me the whole time, apart from a good check-up after she'd fed, and after 10 days in hospital we were allowed home.' **"**

Miscarriage or the death of a baby

In the UK, 1 in 4 pregnancies ends in a miscarriage. Miscarriages usually happen in the first trimester, but late miscarriages can happen up to 24 weeks into pregnancy. You might find out you are miscarrying if you start bleeding, and your team will usually confirm this with a scan. Sometimes your baby has died but you aren't aware until you have a routine scan. This is called a missed miscarriage.

There are different ways for miscarriages to be managed, and the options should be explained to you fully so that you can make a decision. These might include:

- Waiting for your miscarriage to start or progress without any intervention.
- Taking tablets to start a miscarriage and allowing this to progress.
- A surgical procedure, usually under general anaesthetic.

The Miscarriage Association website has lots of information about these options, what will happen during each and the risks and benefits of the different ways of managing a miscarriage.

How you might feel after baby loss

Miscarriage can be unexpected and devastating for women and their partners, and feelings during and afterwards can be wide-ranging, changing and different. According to the Miscarriage Association, the most common feelings around baby loss include feeling:

- Sad and tearful – perhaps suddenly bursting into tears without any obvious trigger.

- Shocked and confused – especially if there were no signs that anything was wrong.

- Numb – you don't seem to have any feelings at all.

- Angry – at fate, at hospital staff, or at others' pregnancy announcements.

- Jealous – especially when seeing other pregnant women and babies.

- Guilty – perhaps wondering if you might have caused the miscarriage (that's very unlikely).

- Empty – a physical sense of loss.

- Lonely – especially if others don't understand.

- Panicky and out of control – feeling unable to cope with everyday life.

Sometimes insensitive care given during a miscarriage can make this worse, but there is growing awareness of the importance of talking about miscarriage, treating women who are miscarrying sensitively and in providing some support services.

NHS services for counselling after miscarriage can be patchy. But if you would like some support following a miscarriage, please see your GP. Private counselling services are available, and there is lots of peer, phone and online support to be found through the Miscarriage Association.

Stillbirth or the death of the baby

Kate's (whose story I shared on page 328) son Thomas died at birth.

> **"** 'I cried a lot, I walked a lot and didn't spend much time at home. Every morning I would put Henry, his twin, in the sling and get out. I think he is still a really empathetic kid to this day because he helped me through all that pain. Over the years that have followed I have been constantly surprised at how many women have lost one of their babies. It seems like such a secret subject. My mother, my aunt, my cousins and friends all had stories that they only felt they could share once I had lost Thomas. I like to talk about him, I tell my children they are one of 4 and the pain of losing him has kind of become a comfort. That I haven't forgotten him, because just the thought of him takes me back to the day when my husband told me he hadn't made it. My 90-year-old neighbour recently told me, with tears in her eyes, that her first son had died and she still thought of him. It was reassuring to know that I would never get over what happened and that was OK.' **"**

After 24 weeks of pregnancy the death of a baby before or during labour is known as a stillbirth. If your baby dies soon after birth, this is known as a neonatal death. If you have just discovered that your baby will be or has been stillborn, you can choose language that feels right for you. Many women prefer to say that their baby has died. And there is no right or wrong or normal way to feel after the devastating news that your baby has died.

As a basic minimum your team should ensure that you are in a private room before, during and after giving birth to your baby. Some maternity units have special bereavement suites and if your midwife doesn't mention it, try to ask about this. You should be assigned an experienced bereavement midwife who can talk you through your options for labour and birth (if your baby dies before it is born), discuss difficult topics such as a post-mortem and a funeral and point you towards lots of sources of support.

You should be given time with your baby after birth, and many units will have special cooling cots to allow you to spend several days with your baby. It can be difficult to decide whether you want to see, hold, photograph, dress and bath your baby. Most couples now decide to do so and I have never spoken to someone who has regretted it.

Only you can decide what feels right for you at the time but, even if you do not wish to see or hold your baby, do ask your midwife to take photographs and make hand and foot-prints. You don't ever have to look at these but they will be there should you change your mind in future.

Checklist

1. Learn more about connecting with your baby if you are separated by reading the tips on page 327. Make sure your partner reads them too, in case you don't remember at the time.
2. If you have a miscarriage or your baby dies, there are lots of places to turn to for help at this very difficult time. SANDS: the Stillbirth and Neonatal Death Charity (www.uk-sands.org) is a good place to start.

Chapter 21

Your No Guilt Pregnancy Plan

It's time to think about what you want and need from your experience of pregnancy, birth and the first weeks with your new baby. Researching, talking and thinking about your plan is almost more important than what it actually says, and yours is going to reflect all the work you've done so far, the decisions you've made and the mindset you want to have.

In this chapter I'll remind you of the key exercises and tools throughout the book, suggesting what will be useful for you. I'll then guide you through what you may want to write down and talk through as you make your plan. The plan itself can be a beautifully formatted document, a series of scrappy Post-it notes stuck to your fridge or simply a prompt for important conversations. The only exception to this is your birth plan, which, as you'll want to share it with your midwife, definitely needs to be written down.

I suggest you make all the plans during your pregnancy. A little time investment now will get you really well set up and save time later. Choose what feels important and right for you from the next pages, remembering that I'm just opening your eyes to options and not telling you what to do.

The outcome

At the end of this chapter you'll have:

1. A short, powerful statement about what you want and need from pregnancy, birth and new motherhood.
2. A more detailed plan for pregnancy, childbirth and beyond, documenting your key decisions and priorities and any important items for your 'to do' list.
3. An 'in labour' checklist to remind you and your partner of what you need to do, to pack, who you need to call and when.
4. Your own little black book of local classes, groups, doulas, feeding support groups and online support.

The big picture – deciding what you want and need

1. Read and do the exercise on page 163 to help you come up with a short statement about what a good birth looks like to you. You'll find the checklists on pages 156, 180, 199, 210, 222 and 253 helpful if you need to read more about birth.
2. Repeat this exercise for pregnancy and the first weeks as a new mother. Take a look at the checklists on pages 38, 52, 96 and 111 (pregnancy) and 270, 283, 294, 320 and 336 (birth) to remind yourself of what might be important to you.
3. Look at your 3 statements and work out what they have in common. Can you write a single statement covering

---

your whole journey to becoming a mother? For example: 'I'll trust myself and my partner but I will always know who to turn to for information, support, compassion and help.'

4. Write your overarching positive statement and your pregnancy, birth and new motherhood statements down on a big piece of paper.

Your pregnancy plan

It's up to you whether it feels useful to write some or all of this plan down, but whether it lives in your head or on paper, working through your pregnancy plan will help you remember which decisions you'll need to make and encourage you to put your wellbeing at the top of your list at this exciting time.

Your body plan

1. Your body is changing. How do you want to feel about your pregnant body and do you need any help to get there? Read the 'body positive' tips on page 22.
2. Eating and drinking in pregnancy can feel like a minefield. Read pages 25–32 for a dietician's advice on cutting through the noise and working out what's right for you. Write down any further research you want to do and any key

decisions you've made about what to avoid or include in your diet.

3. We look at exercise in pregnancy on pages 33–5. What, if anything, are you going to include in your routine? Write down a loose, no-pressure plan for what exercise you'd like to do, and research your local options for classes. Check out www.rebeccaschiller.co.uk/noguilt for helpful videos, DVDs and books if you want to create your own pregnancy exercise plan.

4. Know who to call if you are worried about yourself or your baby during your pregnancy. Write down your maternity helpline number (usually on the front of your maternity notes) and save it in your phone.

Your mind plan

1. Chapter 3 is your go-to resource for all things related to how you might feel in pregnancy. Read it now if you haven't already.

2. If you have a pre-existing mental health condition, consider talking to your midwife, doctor or GP sooner rather than later, to get support and information about how pregnancy and new motherhood might impact on it. Write the plan you have agreed with them down and talk it through with your partner, birth partner and family as appropriate. If you are going to need extra support after the baby is born, start working on that now.

3. Add at least one mindfulness, meditation, relaxation or other self-care exercise into your plan. Commit to how often is realistic for you to do it. Consider making 5 minutes every day for breathing practice (see pages 35, 159 and 274) or a mindfulness activity (see page 282). Can you add a longer piece of self-care (meeting friends, doing a yoga class, getting a massage) once a week?

4. Make a plan to check in with yourself once a month during pregnancy. How are you feeling? What are you happy about and excited by? Can you give these things more space in your life? Is there anything making you feel anxious and, if so, can you or those around you do anything to help? Remember that mood change, anxiety and depression can crop up in pregnancy. See Chapter 3 on getting support.

Not your first baby?

Second/third+ time mothers can find it hard to focus on their new pregnancy or make time for their own needs. You may need to be cunning about timings, but try to find at least 10 minutes, 3 times a week, to take yourself through the tension release exercise on page 46. You may find it helpful to be particularly aware of how your abdomen feels, using your inhalations to connect with your growing baby during this exercise.

Your decisions plan

1. Knowledge is power in pregnancy, so start by reading Chapter 6, which talks you through your key pregnancy decisions.
2. Write down any questions about which tests, screening procedures, antenatal care options are right for you, and add a reminder to your calendar to discuss them at your next midwife's appointment.
3. Write down any key decisions you have made, together with a quick note on why, in case you need reminding later on.

If you've had difficulty conceiving

If you've had a rough ride to pregnancy, had IVF or previous miscarriages, it is very normal to feel anxious about how this pregnancy will go. Check out the support groups on www. rebeccaschiller.co.uk/noguilt and make contact with someone in person or online who has been through pregnancy in similar circumstances to you. Be sure to give the 'Your mind' plan top priority.

Your life plan

1. Make a plan for when to tell your employer and colleagues about your pregnancy. Add in any

adjustments to your work you may need your
employer to make during your pregnancy.

2. Get clued up on your maternity leave and pay rights
   (see page 53–6) and make an appointment to talk
   these through with your employer. If you need
   support, see page 56.

3. Talk to your partner (if you have one) about when
   you might return to work, remembering that you
   don't need to commit to anything now. Write down
   your initial ideas. Look at your finances, career
   goals, childcare options and savings to begin to
   make a plan for a maternity leave that works for
   you. See pages 63–8 for tips on budgeting and
   saving during your pregnancy.

4. Talk to your partner and think through yourself
   the kind of parents you want to be. Are there
   any practicalities, relationship issues or any
   research you need to do to make this a reality? If so,
   work these into your plan. See page 45 for
   suggestions on how to get on the same parenting
   page before your baby is born, and page 59 for
   thinking about how pregnancy might impact on
   your sex life.

5. Add any non-pregnancy stuff you want to achieve,
   enjoy, experience or tick off your list before your
   baby arrives. Think about your home, career goals,
   relationship goals, trips, holidays, skills you want
   to learn. Be realistic about what you have time for
   and can afford, but don't be afraid to make space in
   your plan for things that are nothing to do with
   your baby but will help you hang on to your sense
   of self.

When you've worked through these 5 sections you may need to use the index to get more information on any specific areas, and do visit www.rebeccaschiller.co.uk/noguilt if you need something more in-depth.

High BMI

If you have a high BMI you may find pages 37–8 particularly useful as you make this plan.

Your birth plan

This section is designed to help you work through what a good birth means to you and to translate that into a format your team can work with.

The resulting plan isn't a list of fixed terms and conditions, but a letter to your midwife and/or doctor. It will help them get to know you quickly and build a rapport with you swiftly and easily. It will fill your midwife in on what you've learned about what you need from your environment, the people around you, the things that are important to you and anything you want to avoid during labour and birth. And if your circumstances or your feelings change in labour, it allows your team to suggest the options closest to your original wishes.

'About me' section

Include a couple of the most pertinent facts about you and your partner, so that if you arrive at hospital about to push the baby out, and your midwife can only read the first three sentences of your plan, she has captured the essence of what you need.

Some examples:

'My partner and I are excited about our baby's birth and are having this induction due to my gestational diabetes. We are both deaf and request a BSL interpreter.'

'My partner and I are feeling relaxed and confident and ready to go with the flow. We'd like an active water birth if we can, but know that sometimes plans change. I have a heart condition and my birth plan has been signed off by my consultant and a senior midwife. See page XXX of my notes.'

'I am anxious about giving birth and I have been working hard to help lessen my fears and plan a birth that is OK for me. It's important to me to feel well supported and not alone. I am particularly worried

about tearing and ask for your help in avoiding it if possible and being sensitive to my fear of tearing. Our doula is an important part of our team and has been getting to know us for 6 months.'

Preparing partners

The most useful thing your partner can do is to read this book. You may want to use Post-it notes to suggest the sections you'd really like them to read if they can't manage the whole thing. Make sure they've read the suggestions on using language (see page 178–9), Chapters 9 and 10 on your body and mind during labour, know how to use the BRAIN tool (see page 223), have done the 'What I need from you' exercise (see page 213) with you, and that you have talked through your birth plan with them.

'What I need' section

Remember your 'choosing your birth goal' exercise (page 163)? It's time to share it with your midwife. After telling them who you are, now add what's important to you, no matter what happens during your birth. Keep it short and concentrate on what you need to feel good in and about your baby's birth.

'I want to feel that I am in charge of all decisions, treated kindly and with compassion. My birth plan is important to me, and though I know things might have to change, I will need to feel that you and I did all we could to make it happen and that if plans change we try to keep to the spirit of what I set out below as much as possible.'

'I'm keen to avoid my PTSD triggers and to look back on my birth

feeling it has made me stronger rather than re-traumatized me. This birth plan is designed to help me do that. If it needs to change I'll be anxious and will need your help to avoid feeling panicked.'

'I need to feel that my requests for an epidural are taken seriously and that all is done to enable me to have one as quickly as possible. I'll value your help in managing my contractions until then and will need to know I'm not in this on my own.'

'I need to know that everyone believes, like I do, that I can birth this baby without intervention. I am committed to this home birth and need to stick closely to this well-researched plan unless I feel there is genuine risk to me or my baby.'

Getting your plan respected

If you haven't read Chapter 5 on 'Your Rights', it's time to do so now. Remember to talk through any non-standard decisions you want to make with a senior midwife or doctor before labour. Getting these signed off in advance is really important.

'Labour' section

In the next section of your plan, use bullet points to note any key preferences or decisions. It's not necessary to include things that are standard practice, unless those are particularly important or non-negotiable for you. Instead focus on anything out of the ordinary, or instances where there are a range of options.

Things you may want to include in this section are:

- If you are having a more complex birth and planning to decline any standard care such as continuous foetal monitoring (see page 215).
- If you plan to avoid or limit vaginal examinations (see page 214).
- If you've agreed anything out of the ordinary in advance, such as using the birth pool with a wireless monitor if you are having a VBAC (see page 152), and where this is documented in your notes (see page 345).
- Your plans for pain relief and comfort measures (see pages 145–55). And if you don't want to be offered pain relief unless you request it, note that here too.
- Who will be attending the birth and what their names are (see page 75).
- How important it is to you to be fully informed and make decisions if there's a suggestion that plans change (see page 179).

'Birth' section

In this section you may want to include:

- Whether you would like to give birth in water or not (see page 150).
- If you have any strong feelings about episiotomy (see page 216), or would want a caesarean (see page 232) rather than an assisted birth (page 240).
- If you want to push with your own instincts rather than be directed (or vice versa) (see page 130–131).

- If you have a particular position in mind based on your medical history or your last birth (see page 137).
- If you or your partner want to catch your baby.

Birth planning after trauma

If you've had a traumatic birth or other trauma, making this plan is particularly important. Ensure you and your partner have read Chapter 12, which is dedicated to getting ready for this positive new birth after trauma in the past. The fear release exercise on page 171 may also be really useful to you.

'After birth' section

In this part of the plan it might be useful to include:

- How you would like the third stage to be managed (see page 216).
- How long you would like to leave the cord to pulsate for (see page 220).
- If you have any plans for skin-to-skin, particularly if your birth is likely to be attended by a paediatrician (page 285).
- If you would like uninterrupted time with your baby after birth, a continuation of the quiet, dark and calm environment and any routine measuring, weighing and checking to be done after you have had time to bond with your baby (see page 284).

- If you have any religious or cultural needs that your midwife might not be familiar with, consider including them.
- If you have decided not to breastfeed (see page 315) and do not wish to be asked about this, it may be worth stating this in your birth plan. If you are keen to breastfeed and think you may need or want lots of support (see page 308), add this information to your plan.

This will give you a really clear picture of how you would like things to go if your labour and birth is straightforward and as expected. It will also set out some of the non-negotiable things that you need and expect, however you give birth. I don't think it's necessary for you to include a plan for all eventualities unless it makes you feel much more confident to do this.

In labour checklist

There's lots to remember when you go in to labour, so to help you feel chilled rather than stressed, make a checklist for when you go in to labour. Think about including:

1. Anything you need to add to your birth bag and where it can be found. Remember your notes, money for parking, your camera and any food/drink from the fridge.
2. Who you need to call and when, as well as their numbers. Include taxi companies here if you need them. Remember to talk to your midwife in advance about how best to let them know you are in labour, and when.

3. Any arrangements for other children, along with phone numbers and addresses so your partner doesn't need to check these with you. Add plans for feeding/walking/ caring for pets here too.
4. Anything you need to switch on or off, put in freezer, lock or bins to put out.
5. A reminder to your partner of what you need from them right now. For example, 'Be excited, positive and calm. Ring a friend (secretly) if you feel stressed. Be the guardian of my calm labour space and actively support me in changing position, breathing if it gets tough. Ensure I get what I need, when I need it.'
6. A reminder to yourself to take a moment to notice how you are feeling, focus on your excitement and positivity and use the tools you've learnt to manage any stress or pain. You've got this!

Your afterwards plan

After you've had your baby you'll need to keep things pretty simple for a while. So work through this while you are pregnant, getting set up well in advance so you have what you need and have got into good habits.

Your body

1. Ensure you understand what's normal in terms of symptoms and appearance of a body that's just had a baby (see page 262).

2. Remind yourself to be body positive for your sake and to set an example to your baby. See page 22 for tips, and consider writing some nice things about what your body has done over the last 9 months on your plan and/or on Post-it notes around the house.

3. Make sure you have comfortable, dark clothes, big pants, maternity pads and other essentials for your body (see page 265) in the house by 35 weeks.

4. Decide if and when you might be ready to exercise post-birth and how you are going to do this with a baby in tow. Be ready to be flexible about this if your body has other ideas.

Your mind

1. It's normal to feel strange and emotional after birth. Ensure that you and your partner understand why and what this might look and feel like by reading pages 275–6.

2. Day 4 (ish) (see page 279) can be a tricky day. Make sure you plan a day in bed or on the sofa for this day. Supportive visitors who bring food and don't overstay their welcome only. Remember, it's OK to cancel commitments if you don't feel up to it.

Your decisions

1. Decide on a plan for visitors in advance and get your partner to talk to their family to ensure your

boundaries are respected. Do the same with your family. Consider asking them to bring food, do specific jobs around the house and/or be flexible about when they visit, to respect how you might be feeling.

2. Read pages 296–320 to understand more about your feeding choices. Decide on what goal feels right to you and remember it's OK to change your mind. Read the 'little black book' section below and ensure you have done the 'feeding' part in advance.

3. Work out where your baby is going to sleep and, whatever your plans, read the safe co-sleeping guidelines just in case (see page 278).

Your life

1. Think about what support from a postnatal doula, cleaner, family and friends you will need in the first weeks. Can you ask for any of this as gifts and get any professional support booked in now? See page 276 for ideas.

2. Consider cooking for the freezer in advance so that you and your partner have fewer practical things to do.

3. Go to a local sling meet and learn how to use a stretchy wrap sling. Borrow or buy a sling and practise using it so that you can be hands-free even if your baby doesn't want to be put down.

4. Make a plan for keeping in touch with work and consider whether to put an 'out of office' message on your personal email for the first weeks/months of motherhood.

5. Think and talk about how you and your partner want to protect your relationship after your baby is born. Planning weekly dates is unrealistic at first, but agreeing to open and honest, 'no blame' discussion about tensions and new challenges can be really helpful.

Your little black book

Working out how to get information, support and practical help that's right for you is a big part of this book. www. rebeccaschiller.co.uk/noguilt will signpost you to lots of useful online and in-person groups, as well as the evidence base and helplines that you might need. Don't wait until you need them but spend some time in advance getting clued up on what's out there for you.

1. After making your plan, write down a list of information, professionals, groups, classes and more that you need to make it a reality.
2. Visit www.rebeccaschiller.co.uk/noguilt to begin building a personalized list. Do your own research to add local support, classes, doulas and more to your list.
3. Make sure you include local feeding groups (all the ones in your area, as you don't know which day you may need to visit one), the phone number of an IBCLC (see page 299), a breastfeeding helpline (see page 308) and one of the suggested books about breastfeeding from the resources website if you plan to breastfeed.

Acknowledgements

I promised to bust myths and I'll end with just one more. Writing a book is nothing like having a baby. From idea, to proposal, writing, editing and designing, to holding this finished object takes much longer than nine months. Writing also relies on significantly less bodily fluid but, in my case, a vast amount more swearing.

To get to this point I've leaned heavily on, been boosted, loved, chivvied, reined in and unfailingly supported by so many people. I'd like to thank some of them here, in the hope that they will forget how many drinks I promised to buy them along the way.

My agent, Julia Silk, has represented me and my idea in a way that made everyone believe in us a hundred times more. Julia, when we sat and cried into our lunchtime wine glasses on our first 'date' I knew you were the one. You made this happen. #teamjulia

The incredible Penguin Life team understood my vision for the book so instantly that I relaxed and accidentally dropped the word 'patriarchy' into our first meeting. Nobody flinched and it was clear that I was home. My patient editor, Emily Robertson (and her super efficient assistant Rosanna Forte) managed not to shout when I delivered tens of thousands of extra words and have turned this book into the useful and unbiased guide I hope it is. Julia Murday and Josie Murdoch shaped a brilliant campaign, Sarah Tanat-Jones has brought fabulously real-looking, powerful women to life in her illustrations, Annie Lee copy-edited with skill and insight and Studio Nic&Lou have designed the cover of my dreams.

Experts in their fields have been generous with their time throughout the book and I'm grateful to you all for your help and insight. Significant sections would not have been possible without the brains of Vanessa Christie, Shel Banks, Ashley MacDonald and Adele Hug.

Elizabeth Prochaska, Maria Booker, Rebecca Brione, Rachael Evans and all the trustees and supporters of Birthrights have dedicated so much to our charity because they believe that all women matter in childbirth. It's a belief we share with many midwives, doctors, healthcare professionals and doulas who listen to women and support their right to have agency over their own bodies. It's an honour to be able to thank you here and to give a special mention to Maddie McMahon, Milli Hill, Jessica James, Bridget Baker, Cathy Warwick, Kay Hardie, Angela Barry, Mars Lord, Maisie Hill, the BPAS team, Carolyn Johnston, Naomi Delap, Pascale Hunter, Sheena Byrom, Rebecca Moore and Emma Svanberg.

My friends have kept me going and focused at a time when it would have been easy not to. Amy, Anna, Catherine, Clare, Joanna and Lorna – I promise to do the same for you. My parents have put in some serious grandparenting to help me meet my deadline and also gifted/cursed me with the genetic material that made it seem like a good idea in the first place.

My husband Jared, and our children Sofya and Arthur (and our ever-expanding brood of semi-useful animals) deserve an apology for all the weekends they were evicted so that I could write in peace and for the half-crazed grumpy woman they've had to deal with over the past eighteen months. I can only offer my eternal gratitude to them for continuing somehow to love and believe in me even on those days when I stopped brushing my teeth and hair.

Finally and most importantly, I want to thank the women, people and families who welcomed me into their lives and births as a doula, sharing their strength, vulnerability, joy and pain. And the many others who gave their most intimate of stories to these pages. You are the heart of this book.

Index

pumps, 2, 66, 300, 301
and sex, 61
sharing the load, 304
and sleep, 278
stretchy wrap slings, 292
underdeveloped breasts, 310
breasts, 267
colostrum, 15, 260, 267, 300,
313–14, 328
enlargement, 11, 60, 66, 225,
260, 264, 267
hypoplasia, 310
insufficent glandular tissue
(IGT), 310
inverted nipple shape, 310
leaking, 15, 20, 267, 269, 326
mastitis, 312
milk, 260, 266, 267, 268, 279,
300–301, 309–11
nipple cream, 66
nipples, darkening of, 267
sensitivity, 11, 60, 100
underdeveloped, 310
breathing
labour, 35, 159, 174–6
newborns, 288
breathing practice, 280, 293
alternate nostril breathing,
274, 293
labour, 35, 118, 159,
174–6, 237
yoga, 35–6, 280
breech babies, 17, 242–4
*British Journal of Obstetrics and
Gynaecology*, 270
butterfly mask of pregnancy, 100

caesareans, 73, 74, 77, 146, 149,
193, 195–9, 226
breastfeeding, 297, 299, 315
breathing, 176, 237
calm playlist, 169
crash, 239–40
early labour, 116, 162
elective, 18, 74, 116,
146, 182, 183, 195–9,
206, 207
emergency, 94, 197–9,
232–40, 243
epidurals, 149
and exercise, 269
going home, 291
high risk, 230
pain relief, 238–9, 259
personalization, 234
placenta praevia, 109
pre-eclampsia/HELLP
syndrome, 108
pre-labour, 124
risks and benefits, 197
and size of baby, 105–6
skin-to-skin, 195–6,
199, 237
transverse labour, 244
VBAC (vaginal birth after
caesarean), 71, 79, 152,
208–10
calcium, 26, 85, 268
calm triggers, 167–70, 205
cannulas, 78, 79, 147, 235, 251
carpal tunnel, 98
catheter, 132
cats, 86, 99